C000017351

Medicines Management

Medicines Management

Edited by

Rhona Panton and Stephen Chapman

Department of Medicines Management
Keele University, UK

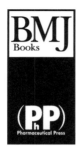

© BMJ Books and Pharmaceutical Press 1998
BMJ Books is an imprint of the BMJ Publishing Group

All rights reserved. No part of this publication may be reproduced,
stored in a retrieval system, or transmitted, in any form or by any
means, electronic, mechanical, photocopying, recording and/or
otherwise, without the prior written permission of the publishers.

First published in 1998
by BMJ Books, BMA House, Tavistock Square,
London WC1H 9JR
and
Pharmaceutical Press, 1 Lambeth High Street, London SE1 7JN

British Library Cataloguing in Publication Data

A catalogue record for this book is available from the
British Library

ISBN 0-7279-1274-7

Typeset, printed and bound in Great Britain by
Latimer Trend & Company Ltd, Plymouth

Contents

Contributors

Alison Blenkinsopp
Director of Education and Research
Department of Medicines Management
Keele University
Keele, UK

Colin Bradley
Professor of General Practice
Department of General Practice
University College Cork
Ireland

Stephen Chapman
Professor of Prescribing Studies
Department of Medicines Management
Keele University
Keele, UK

Wendy Clark
Lecturer and MTRAC Drug Information Pharmacist
Department of Medicines Management
Keele University
Keele, UK

Naaz Coker
Fellow
The King's Fund
11–13 Cavendish Square
London, UK

David Dickinson
Principal Consultant
Consumation
53 Hosack Road
London, UK

Alan Earl-Slater
Senior Lecturer Health Economics
Department of Medicines Management
Keele University
Keele, UK

Mike Fisher
General Practitioner, Stoke-on-Trent, UK
and Chairman
Midland Therapeutic Review and Advisory Committee

Ray Fitzpatrick
Director of Pharmacy
North Staffs Hospital NHS Trust and Senior Lecturer Pharmacy
Practice
Department of Medicines Management
Keele University
Keele, UK

Martin Frischer
Senior Lecturer Health Services Research
Department of Medicines Management
Keele University
Keele, UK

Elena Grant
Regional Drug Information Pharmacist
West Midlands Region
Good Hope Hospital NHS Trust
Sutton Coldfield, UK

John Mucklow
Consultant Clinical Pharmacologist
North Staffs Hospital NHS Trust and
Senior Lecturer Clinical Pharmacology and Therapeutics
Department of Medicines Management
Keele University
Keele, UK

Jeff Norwood
Consultant in Public Health Medicine
Walsall Health Authority and Lecturer Public Health
Department of Medicines Management
Keele University
Keele, UK

Rhona Panton
Emeritus Professor of Medicines Management
Department of Medicines Management
Keele University
Keele, UK

Ian Purves
Head of Sowerby Centre
Sowerby Centre for Health Informatics at Newcastle Primary
Care Development Centre
University of Newcastle upon Tyne
Newcastle upon Tyne, UK

Kate Tunna
Tutor, Centre for Ethics
Department of General Practice
University of Birmingham Medical School
Birmingham, UK

Tom Walley
Professor of Pharmacology and Therapeutics
Department of Pharmacology and Therapeutics
University of Liverpool
Liverpool, UK

Preface

New medicines are now the subject of everyday debate. Barely a week passes without the media reporting a new and wonderful medicine superior in every respect to those it replaces. Often such reports are followed by patients or patient associations reporting that health authorities cannot or will not pay for the new product. Patients are then interviewed explaining how greatly they would benefit from its use and the spokesperson for the health authority then has to justify the decision. Evidence of inequity in the system is shown when it becomes clear that should this patient choose to move 50 miles down the road, a different health authority would pay for the medicine. Such encounters rarely address the wider issues of the strength of the clinical evidence, the way the price was set, or the other services that would have to be foregone to pay for it.

This book is designed to explore all the issues that should be considered in the decision making process, and so to ensure that decisions are fair, justifiable, and shared with patients.

Some of the work described in this book has been developed in one health region in the United Kingdom, the West Midlands, which we believe has the potential for national application. New and cost effective drugs should be introduced into practice as widely and quickly as possible. Those of little proven benefit should not.

The first three chapters give the perspective on medicines usage of a patient, an ethicist, and a general practitioner.

David Dickinson sets out the dilemma of the consumer as patient and citizen, and makes a strong case for sharing information with patients at the earliest possible time. The ethical framework for making decisions on resource allocation in a publicly funded service is addressed by Kate Tunna in chapter 2 which reminds us that the practice of evidence based medicine is also an ethical issue. The role of the GP in medicines management is explored by Colin

Bradley in chapter 3 which makes recommendations for better management of prescribing in primary care.

The fourth chapter then sets the scene for a considered approach to medicines management by reviewing the rise in the drug bill and the factors that affect it. It reviews Government policies for medicines use and worldwide methods of controlling their cost.

The next three chapters then consider how to assess the evidence. The basis of evidence based medicine—clinical trials and their interpretation—is set out in chapter 5 by John Mucklow and Wendy Clark who discuss the sources of evidence, and review the different types of trial design and the fundamental points of importance in their interpretation. The tools of the trade in prescribing analysis are discussed in chapter 6 which lists the databases available and discusses the problems inherent in the interpretation of such data. It describes the various methods of prescribing analysis and give examples of their use. Chapter 7 discusses the need to address wider issues than drug acquisition costs including cost–benefit analysis, measurement of the burden of disease, and opportunity costs. This chapter also considers the patient's agenda.

The agencies available to give further help on decision making are set out by Tom Walley in chapter 8 which gives an excellent summary of all UK organisations involved in giving specialist support to medicines management.

Getting research into practice is the subject of chapter 9. This chapter describes a West Midlands success, a regional GP committee which evaluates the evidence and empowers GPs to make recommendations to their colleagues for the use of new medicines. It also describes practice based prescribing support and the work of Medical Audit Advisory Groups in prescribing analysis.

Educational outreach has the potential to ensure that all prescribers can be visited in a short period of time and given a structured, evidence based message to implement research findings and change prescribing practice. This is the subject of chapter 10.

Hospital based methods of medicines management are discussed in chapter 11 which considers how they can be adapted and developed to systems management for a coordinated approach.

Finally, a short summary reminds readers of the issues identified in the book as essential to better medicines management and briefly considers a fourth hurdle.

Editing this book has been a pleasure and the task made easy by the willing contributions of all our chapter editors and supporting

writers. Thanks to all of them. Separate and very special thanks are also due to Elly Reeve who has master minded the whole enterprise by devising workplans, encouraging everyone to stick to them, and for a big contribution in the final presentation. Wendy Clark has given a willing and expert contribution to nearly every chapter. Thanks also to Martin Kendall for a valuable contribution to chapter 5, to Jo Lockett and Lynne Nadin, our data analysts, to Judith Misson for checking references and to Marie Richardson for typing the script.

Rhona Panton
Stephen Chapman

1 That's my medicine: medicines management for consumers and citizens

DAVID DICKINSON

All the medicines management in the world will not help the National Health Service (NHS) if people who indirectly pay for and ultimately take the medicines will not buy into it. The biggest problems are gaps in attitudes: first a gap between patients and professionals and second the gap within us all between consumer and citizen. People have dual attitudes to publicly funded medicines: one is a citizen's, public interest attitude that tolerates rationing; the other, is the hunger of *patient as consumer* to get the right treatment immediately at the time it is needed. In the first state of mind, people's support for the NHS leads them to understand its dilemmas and put up with its compromises. In the second state, patient consumers (or often carers) will see drug rationing through different eyes, and will often start to see the NHS (whether represented by their general practitioner (GP) or their health authority) as an enemy withholding treatment. Their sympathies and those of patient groups start to be more with the pharmaceutical industry, which has developed the treatments for them. The industry naturally is beginning to spend time and money getting closer to patients and putting its messages in their language. I suggest that the public sector also needs to do this too.

The objectives of this chapter are to recognise four phenomena and take steps to remedy them:

1   The gap between professionals and lay people.
2   The gap between citizens and consumers.

1

3 The NHS as a mean spirited enemy.
4 Communicating with patients who don't believe you.

The gap between patients and professionals

There is a gap between patients and professionals. The two groups think differently about illness; they make different decisions about treatment based on the same facts. More and more research shows the disparity, and that it may be particular or general. For example, in one study people with multiple sclerosis rated relative disability of lesser importance than doctors did.[1] In the work of Dianne Berry, what patients want to know about medicines (in two words—side effects) differs markedly from what doctors want to tell them.[2] There is no great shame or surprise about this. We are waking up to the fact that health professionals—with several years of formal training on top of a university education, with jobs, and in reasonable health—think differently to the rest of the population who come to them for advice because they are sick.

One initiative, *From compliance to concordance*,[3] encapsulates the difference between the two groups. The concept of concordance rejects the idea that patients behave irrationally when they do not take medicines as professionals would expect (that is, rationally). Instead it recognises two groups of people—patients and professionals—approaching the health care transaction with two separate rationales. This expert working group's report stresses the need for health professionals involved in medicine taking to elicit, examine, and share the patient's rationale about medicinal decision making. Professionals and patients need to forge a *therapeutic alliance* against disease; the resulting agreement is summed up as concordance, not merely compliance.

Why does concordance matter for medicines management?

- It matters because the best policy in the world will fail to provide value and efficiency if the ultimate managers of medicines—the patients who take them—are not involved, their motives understood and examined, and recruited to a therapeutic alliance—in the cause of better medicine management.

- It matters because patients in some areas of the country and with certain illnesses are beginning to perceive the NHS at local level as a villain, rather than a hero: as a withholder, not a provider.
- It matters because, if the NHS fails to make allies of these patients, there is the pharmaceutical industry that will be happy to fill the gap, via the media or patient groups. That may not be undesirable—unless it excludes or bypasses the NHS.

Citizens and consumers: people as well as patients

There is another gap, as well as that between professional and patient. It is the gap that exists within each of us, between our private and public needs—between the consumer of medicines or health care, and the citizen of the UK.

On one level the relationship is simple: you become a consumer of medicines or services when you are ill; the rest of the time you're a citizen with a citizen's interest in the NHS. When you are on a waiting list, you worry (as a consumer) about how long you will wait. But there is also an issue of how many people are on waiting lists. This is not a worry to the consumer in us, but an issue of public concern.

Evidence for this public concern comes from the King's Fund. In its annual review of health care was an article, "Public opinion and the NHS", which seems to show increasing public gloom about various aspects of the NHS.[4] This was not simply consumer pressure; the authors noted that recent hospital patients were *less* likely to be dissatisfied with the running of the NHS. They speculated that public dissatisfaction might be a function of media images of the NHS and perceptions of how much was being spent:

> In Britain there ... seem to be strong associations between priorities for public spending, levels of dissatisfaction with the NHS and the generosity or otherwise of the annual public spending round. In short, the public appears to want to see sustained levels of reasonably generous funding for the NHS.

They also warned that, whether real or media fuelled,

> ... the fact that there appears to be a growing disillusionment with specific health services might, in the longer term, undermine support for the basic principles of the NHS.

3

One way of reading this fascinating research (of which this is the barest summary) is that passionate, private, consumer concerns about the state of the NHS are (for the moment) allayed when patients actually get treated. As most of us are not patients at any particular time, they are outnumbered by more generalised public, citizen style concerns about the decline in values of the NHS as filtered through the media. This may help to explain why people have not taken to the streets over the NHS: passion at that level rarely arises from liberal public concern, but from private personal grievance. That sort of grievance appears to be reduced in hospital patients, who (crudely put) learn to love the system. Consumer and citizen concerns do not coincide. In issues of medicines provision, however, there is not just public concern. Private grievance may arise in people denied medicines, especially if media coverage starts to fan the flames. Could the management of medicines make a public enemy of the NHS?

The NHS as a mean spirited enemy

If I am part of a focus group or survey sample, and I am asked about the needs of the NHS drugs budget, I might react in one of two ways. One is to say: "Yes well of course I understand that the NHS budget is not a bottomless pile of gold and so, yes, I suppose that some sort of rationing is inevitable." That sounds suitably pompous and wise. The other is to say: "But I *need* my medicines. I'm a taxpayer. I've *paid* for them." That may sound shrill, even selfish. But both voices are mine: they are the voices of the citizen and the consumer. The difference may be no more than illness.

Suppose an older relative of mine falls sick with dementia. Spending limits that I may support as a prudent taxpayer begin to look different. The GP's refusal to prescribe a given medicine will make a real, very practical difference to my life and my relative's life. Suppose that the GP duly explains that her hands are tied by local prescribing policy. If the medicine is one that I know for a fact from the newspapers to be a miraculous cure for Alzheimer's disease, my resentment will start to heat up. If I then discover that the medicine in question would be available in a neighbouring health authority, my mood is likely to reach a rolling boil. If I am enterprising, I take the story to the papers myself, desperate to try to secure drug treatment through publicity—and a sensible, public

spirited person has flipped over and become a loose consumerist cannon.

It is that easy to make enemies of the people. In this state of mind, the NHS is a villain. The perception of the miserly NHS may be spreading to the people who are well. Work soon to be published by Vikki Entwistle of the NHS Centre for Research and Dissemination at York and by Angela Coulter of the King's Fund looked at materials for the general public on treatment choices. People looking at those generated by the NHS had suspicions that can be paraphrased as "well they would say that, wouldn't they?". They didn't trust the NHS's motives for recommending certain treatments above others.

If you thought that the NHS had a special place in the hearts of British people, you would be right. But if anybody thought that this special place was inviolable, it looks as if they were wrong.

Based on misconceptions

You will have noticed that the anecdote of alienation I outlined rests on three misconceptions. If you can address those misconceptions, you are on the way to solving the associated problems.

First, there is the murky business of whose decision it is—to prescribe or not to prescribe? A GP is expected to give out the bad news that a drug will not be prescribed; it is only natural in that situation to stress the role of others in making these unpopular decisions. After all the GP has to keep alive a relationship with her patients; and a relationship is something the health authority does not have. Second, the effectiveness of drugs is misunderstood in two directions: the limits of what they can do and what constitutes effectiveness. It has been said that there are only two media stories about medicines: killer drugs and miracle cures. Certainly the finer points of cost–benefit analysis rarely figure in press coverage of medicines, new or not. What is more, the media's interest is usually in an individual's story—anecdotal in every sense. Where media articles are compressed, what tends to stay in the memory is a headline—which is not usually written by the journalist who wrote the story. The third misconception is that the system of NHS prescribing is, deep down, somehow fair or equitable. The press is full of people who would have got more suitable (and more expensive) treatment if they had only lived down the road. The

British Medical Association has called the phenomenon "postcode rationing", and it is still newsworthy for two reasons: because it is not (yet) universally known and because it is so unfair.

To tackle these misconceptions, purchasers need to see that they have a relationship with the public (whether they like it or not), and that making it a good relationship relies on good communication. Tackling the misconceptions above is just part of communicating what managers of medicines are doing. But communication is a two way process. After contact with patients, it may be necessary for purchasers to ask whether their agenda is the right one.

Communicating with patients: why they don't believe you

Many patient groups view evidence based medicine as having limited value. Why? The radical patient agenda argues that trials only answer the questions that professionals have put. It is only recently that quality of life measures have begun to be introduced into clinical trials (see chapter 7), and it is still not usual. For drugs with dramatic benefits to the quality of a patient's life, a trial that measures only clinical outcomes will miss the point. For example, it was the cost of erythropoietin that worried most medicines managers on its introduction, although the truly dramatic difference that the drug made to patients' lives, changed the picture. We have already seen, above, how different patients' and physicians' views on multiple sclerosis can be. Patient friendly decisions can be made only after patient input. There are also clinical reasons for patient centred measures in trials. For instance, patients will stop taking a medicine that has sufficiently unpleasant side effects. If the trials do not record their reasons, or fail to ask the patients' views about side effects, the drug will appear to fail in trials—without its therapeutic effect having been actually put to the test. In the name of high quality evidence, patient defined outcomes should be considered in every trial, otherwise the evidence base on which decisions about new drugs are taken will continue to have nothing in it for patients. Evidence based medicines will alienate them.

Views such as this need to be taken on board by the new Commission for Health Improvement and the National Institute

for Clinical Excellence, as well as by every purchaser of medicines. Who are the medicines designed to benefit? Patients, naturally. Where are the views of those notional beneficiaries in the research, interpretation, and decision making about medicines? Usually, nowhere. There is already a Standing Advisory Group on Consumer Involvement in the NHS Research and Development Programme (PO Box 1629, Hassocks, BN6 8EP). But there is some way to go before either citizens or consumers take a full part in decision making. Patients do not just need to be told about the decisions made for them in the health service. As with concordance, we need to forge a new culture in which consumers and citizens are part of the decision making committees and groups, and in which it is natural that patient groups, consumer groups, and committed individuals should take part in the process. They have a distinctive point of view and a legitimate interest in how public money is spent and what decisions are taken.

Purchasers need a relationship with patients

A GP has a relationship with patients. The pharmaceutical industry is busy cultivating one. Makers of prescription drugs do not formally have direct contacts with patients (while prescription drug advertising to patients is still illegal), but conferences and meetings on the theme of "patient partnership" are big sellers, and the industry funds or supports ever more vocal patient groups. There are strong common interests between consumers and industry. For example, people with multiple sclerosis, or their carers, want interferon-β to be available as a choice. The manufacturers want it too. When the makers of one brand, Schering Health Care Limited, estimate that only 20 or 30 health authorities are funding "realistic levels of the drug to realistic numbers of patients,"[5] it is hard to tease out industry marketing and patient advocacy.

So the doctor has a relationship; the manufacturer is cultivating a relationship. Where is the purchaser in all this? If a medicine is not prescribed, it is in the interests of the health authority to get in and explain why not—to create a relationship with the public. That is what the other players have already done. Otherwise, the message received by consumers is of a decision by faceless bureaucrats in grey suits, based entirely on cost. That is a quick route to loss of public confidence.

Purchasers need to explain medicines and the system

Prescribers and the pharmaceutical industry have put their case forcefully in debates about rationing, but a purchaser's role is harder to understand. We have already seen that effectiveness of medicines means different things to different people. Patients may fairly claim that research evidence does not usually aim at meeting patients' needs, but at answering clinical questions. Purchasers need to join the move to help people interpret evidence, and to start encouraging and acting on research that addresses patients' needs. These actions will not only help a responsible authority to explain its decisions in context, but will also keep decision makers in touch with patients' concerns, and lengthen and strengthen that relationship.

Getting messages across

Practically speaking, how do we create relationships and put messages across? We do it in the same way as the other players do it.

- **Collect public opinion to act on:** qualitative research may be most helpful. Innovations such as citizens' juries—in which people are collected for several days and asked to hear the case for issues such as rationing in the NHS—are achieving interesting results under the sponsorship of groups such as the Institute of Public Policy Research and the King's Fund. But they are still very expensive to mount. Focus groups are a cheaper alternative, although they are vulnerable to being hijacked by one or two vociferous individuals. But they do allow the patients' agenda to emerge.

- **Keep up contacts with patient groups:** listening as well as talking to them. Two bodies with excellent data on patient and self-help groups are the College of Health (0181 983 1225) and the Help for Health Trust (01962 849100). The Local NHS Health Information Service (0800 66 55 44) will have details, too.

- **Expand patient communication:** web sites, leaflets, videos and newsletters can all help to put your case. Communication needs to be not just in plain language, but to address the right areas. The most effective communications involve consumers by piloting and auditing materials before publication. My own

consultancy specialises in this field; the Centre for Health Information Quality (01962 863511) keeps databases of good practice and experienced practitioners in drafting patient materials, and its referrals are free to the NHS and patient groups.

- **Cultivate health journalists:** on local and national media (radio and television as well as press); have case studies and stories up your sleeve. Remember in this context that journalists like true stories, of individuals, children, and traumatic tales (though they are permitted to have happy endings). Try to talk one to one with journalists—it is easier to make sure that they have understood you—and do not assume that they know what you are talking about.
- **Hold public meetings:** perhaps in conjunction with patient groups to help attendance and manage the mood.

There is an extensive literature on consumer involvement in health care,[6] but these suggestions are more pragmatic. In effect, they add up to good public relations. But that doesn't mean window dressing. Ultimately, public involvement in management decisions is the only way to create a sustainable relationship between the British public and the health service that is funded from its taxes. Until then, think of my suggestions as emergency bridges across the gaps between citizens, consumers, and a health service in danger of becoming the enemy.

1 Rothwell PM, McDowell Z, Wong CK, Dorman PJ. Doctors and patients don't agree: cross-sectional study of patients' and doctors' perceptions and assessments of disability in multiple sclerosis. *BMJ* 1997;**314**:1580–3.
2 Berry DC, Michas IC, Gillie T, Forster M. What do patients want to know about their medicines, and what do doctors want to tell them? *Psychol Health* 1997;**12**:467–80.
3 Marinker M, ed. *From compliance to concordance: achieving shared goals in medicine taking.* London: Royal Pharmaceutical Society of Great Britain and Merck Sharp & Dohme Limited, 1997.
4 Mulligan JA, Judge K. Public opinion and the National Health Service. Health Care United Kingdom 1996–9. *King's Fund annual review of health policy.* London: King's Fund, 1997:123–37.
5 Wallace ME, quoted in "Patients, drug firms oppose rationing". *Patient* November 1997;1. London.
6 King's Fund. *User involvement in health care, reading list No 5.* London: King's Fund, September 1997.

2 The ethics of prescribing

KATE TUNNA

This chapter starts with a brief discussion of the central role of philosophy in medicine and goes on to examine, in particular, the ethical principles that underlie the prescribing of medicines in primary care. These considerations underpin the ethical framework for decision making, described in this chapter, to which general practitioners can appeal in clarifying their obligation to prescribe not only the most effective medicine for the treatment of the patient's ailment, but also the least expensive. Essentially this chapter is addressing the question of clinical and cost effectiveness from an ethical perspective. It will be argued that, in prescribing medicines, in addition to directly addressing the two pressing clinical issues, "Does this drug work in the treatment of this particular condition" and "Is it safe?", responsible medical practitioners must also consider cost effectiveness in the form of the question, "Is it worth it?" Doctors, as autonomous moral agents, are not at liberty to prescribe in ways that necessitate excessive expenditures that are expected to result in no added therapeutic benefit over and above the cheaper available alternatives, provided those alternatives still satisfy the criteria of clinical effectiveness and safety.

The ethical framework proposed in this chapter is a further application of a previous model developed by Heather Draper and Kate Tunna for the Nuffield Institute for Health, Leeds.[1]

Philosophy in medicine

In their classic text, *A philosophical basis of medical practice*, Pellegrino and Thomasma examine the sometimes fraught relationship between philosophy and medicine (page 9).[2]

Medicine and philosophy oscillate about each other like strands of a complex double helix of the intellect. They are intermittently drawn together by their immersion in human existence and driven apart by their often opposing pre-occupations with that existence.

Practising clinicians often complain that moral philosophy, of which ethics is a branch, has a poor understanding of the practical everyday problems raised by health and illness. Similarly, ethicists will argue that many a medical decision is made without even the slightest effort to clarify the problem or justify the decision by appeal to ethical theory and principles.

Tenuous though the nature of this relationship may be, this chapter is based on the premise that the practice of medicine is first and foremost a moral endeavour, undertaken in order that people who already are, or who may find themselves in, wounded states can be reassured, relieved, or benefited in some way. It is precisely because health care systems are created and maintained for the benefit of society and its members that the delivery of such care is fundamentally moral in nature. In further recognition of its philosophical basis, it is important not to forget that medicine operates through an intense human relationship in which doctor and patient must negotiate a process of value laden decision making which has, as its aim, the curing or amelioration of illness, and the promotion of health. Good medicine is defined by good ethics. By admitting ethics into their practice clinicians uphold their responsibility for illuminating, examining, and clarifying their everyday activity.

Undoubtedly a discipline in its own right, with its own traditions, theories, empiricism, and methods, applied ethics becomes most interesting when it leaves the misty flats of abstraction and busies itself among the thorny day to day issues of clinical life. Clinicians are constantly wondering about what should be done or what ought to be done in a given situation. Medicine, as it is both taught and practised, is case orientated and even the youngest of students is encouraged to consider the merits of each individual case—what is happening to this patient, at this time, and in this situation. Indeed, to be an effective healer, the clinician must take account of the particularities of the patient in the context of his or her life. However, as Veatch[3] pointed out long ago, if the ethical issue or problem in each case is treated as something entirely fresh or

entirely novel, apart from being overwhelmed by detail, clinicians will be denied the opportunity to understand general principles of ethics through which they can distinguish categories of problems and generate categories of solutions for themselves. Viewed in this light, ethics offers nothing different from any other set of theoretical propositions—be they physiological, anatomical, or biochemical. Solutions to ethical problems are grounded in ethical theory and principles in the same way that solutions to blood pressure difficulties are grounded in theories of cardiovascular haemodynamics.

So, in this chapter which seeks, first and foremost, to offer an ethical framework for prescribing decisions, a brief description of ethical principles is included in the hope that it will aid the clinician's attempt to work through ethical problems of prescribing in today's resource limited environment. To be effective these principles require that their application is supported by the traditional tools of philosophy—critical reflection and reasoned analysis. The framework, which has previously been applied to purchasing in the NHS,[1] can be used to assist doctors to reach justifiable prescribing decisions in different situations, while still acknowledging the unique attributes of the patient and his or her particular difficulties.

Four ethical principles in health care decision making

In Western health care systems, four main principles of ethics—non-maleficence, beneficence, autonomy, and justice— have been widely adopted as the structural basis of ethical decision making in health care delivery. It is necessary to point out, however, that, although these principles may be defended by some,[4,5] others[6] reject them on the grounds that they result in a watered down conception of the moral demands of life, lacking both substance and bite. Despite this criticism, their particular usefulness, it seems, may be found in their capacity to transcend cultural, political, and religious precepts and thereby offer health care providers a broadly acceptable foundation upon which to build their ethical decisions.

In the next section, the four principles will be described briefly and their relevance discussed for GPs operating in resource limited prescribing contexts.

The combined principle of non-maleficence and beneficence

These two principles are probably best viewed together. Non-maleficence refers to the specific obligation of not inflicting harm, whereas beneficence refers to the wider aims of attempting to prevent and remove harm as well as to promote good. Needless to say, difficulties arise in how harm and benefit can be determined and by whom. Disagreement here can create *ethical tension* in the doctor–patient relationship in which the two parties are at odds in deciding how best to meet the patient's best interests. This challenge of balancing harms against benefits is made harder by resource limitation, because, under those circumstances, doctors have to demonstrate not only that they have prevented harm, removed harm, and promoted good, but also that they have shown that their spending was not only likely to result in clinical benefit, but was also cost effective. Spending in ways that are cost ineffective may limit the amount of potential overall benefit that could be conferred on a given patient population. This is *not* to say that the obligation to promote benefit is attenuated in any way in a resource limited context. Benefit must still be maximised but, at the same time, there must be a strict accounting of every penny spent.

In summary, the principles of non-maleficence and beneficence dictate that it is morally irresponsible either to purchase or to prescribe treatments and therapies of dubious value, those that appear to do no good, and those that actually do harm. This is wrong whether or not we are faced with the problem of limited resources. When resources are limited, however, cost effectiveness also has to be taken into account in calculating best interests, because the investment of scarce monies may result in depriving some patients of much needed treatments, thereby causing them harm. Implicit in this last statement is the recognition that resource limited conditions may constrain the autonomy, not only of the practitioner, but also of the patient.

The principle of autonomy

Autonomy or self determination is born out of moral responsibility and manifests itself in three ways: freedom of will, freedom of thought, and freedom of action.[1] In a prescribing context this means that doctors are free to think through clinical

problems for themselves, use their knowledge and skill to fathom possible solutions, and then to choose how they will act—what they will do about the problems at hand. This freedom imposes significant responsibilities and choices can be troublesome for health professionals who must choose between different courses of action, some of which can be expected to result in good outcomes, whereas others might bring about less desirable ends. At all times, upholding their moral responsibility obliges clinicians to act in such a way that they will, to the best of their belief, choose the course of action that will maximise benefit and minimise harm. So, although doctors are autonomous in the sense that they are in possession of and capable of exercising their free will, their freedom is limited by the ethical imperative of enhancing human good.

The choice of a pharmaceutical product, for example, in the treatment of a patient's condition, can be very difficult to make against the pressure of manufacturers' competing claims. Clinicians are besieged, one might even say overwhelmed, by choices that offer new and better therapeutic solutions to clinical problems. But choice, in and of itself, does not enhance autonomy. This only occurs if the choice about which we are speaking gives us greater control over our lives. The choice of a new and apparently improved medicine will only increase the control in our lives if it is likely to result in greater therapeutic benefit than all other available alternatives, and if it fails to impose unnecessary financial burden, which could mean that others will be deprived.[1]

Whether or not to prescribe a more costly alternative, for whatever reason—manufacturers' or patients' pressure or request by hospital colleagues—is a relatively problem free decision when resources are plentiful, but when they are not ethical *pressures* will constrain autonomy. Under conditions of limited resource, everybody involved in the system—from purchasers to patients—has a responsibility to protect the fund, to purchase, to prescribe, and to consume responsibly and judiciously. It should not be forgotten that the monies used to pay for medicines and therapies belong to the patients in a given community; they are paid for through the collection of taxes, an obligation from which no one can be exempted. To prescribe in ways that are inefficient, either clinically or economically, is to waste tax monies; this thereby represents a betrayal of the trust of those who have contributed.

14

The principle of justice

Bearing in mind that health care monies derived from taxation are held in trust, contributors to the purse may rightfully expect that those charged with the responsibility of distributing those monies—be it as a result of purchasing or prescribing—will do so in as fair and just a manner as possible. This commitment to "distributive justice" is a significant element in the obligation of all health care providers, not merely to avoid harm and do good, but to maximise benefit and minimise harm. Distributive justice is the mechanism through which benefits (health care) and burdens (taxation) are distributed fairly in society and the concept assumes major importance, not to mention unbearable tension, in circumstances of limited resource. How do we decide who gets what when there is not enough to go around? The answer to this very difficult question requires consideration of the material principles of justice.[7] A thorough treatment of these is beyond the scope of this chapter; however, four will be discussed briefly because each has at least some impact on health care delivery in the general practice setting.

Everyone should be given the same

In general practice, giving the *same* to patients really means acknowledging a bottom line below which no one's care descends. This encapsulates the notion of a decent minimum standard of health care available to all and it requires that people with similar illnesses be treated, by and large, in similar ways. Each patient with illness X will receive the best available alternative in terms of clinical and cost efficiency, individual considerations aside. In addition to pharmacological treatment, giving the same also means that doctors as professionals will treat all patients with equal respect and concern.

Benefit should be distributed according to need

Need, as a means of distributing benefit, accords well with our everyday experience of the moral life. People in need generate our sympathy and compassion irrespective of how their need arose, causing us to dig deep into our pockets to ease their plight. This is the case with health care in that we expect and generally would wish that the most severely ill—those most in need—would receive greater assistance than others. Goodwin[8]

15

discusses equity in health care as being centred upon need (page 17):

> Equity is about services being needs-based. People in equal need should have equal access to services and those whose needs are greater should be targeted to receive proportionately more of whatever resources are available.

Although this sentiment strikes one as entirely fair, the problem with it is only too apparent, namely defining need and, further, distinguishing between needs and wants. Therapies such as cosmetic surgery, infertility treatment, or the prescribing of cholesterol lowering medicines to support a grossly unhealthy lifestyle are all questionable in terms of whether they respond to genuine health care *need*. When need is defined in relation to anticipated benefit, costly interventions for people in persistent vegetative state, for example, might be denied. Need may also be denied if it requires the clinician to act beyond the limit of the law, such as providing cannabis for a patient with intractable nausea or deliberately ending the life of someone who requests euthanasia.

Even when need is clearly defined and easily recognised, it still may go unmet because resources simply are not plentiful enough or they are not distributed in such a way as to answer all existing health needs. In these circumstances, severity of need may be calculated using some index of morbidity and mortality if treatment is withheld or limited, or potential health gain if treatment is applied. Worth remembering is the fact that needs are identified as being more pressing when the distributor of the resource, namely the GP in the present discussion, meets the patient face to face. The intensity of this relationship coupled with the complexities of the clinical encounter, as well as the doctor's unique knowledge of the patient, may render him or her less able to deny the needs claimed by the patient. So although "Health of The Nation" targets, for example, may respond to perceived population needs, individual clinicians may find themselves operating in ways that run counter to those aims.

Benefit should be distributed according to personal effort

The notion of people having a pre-existing moral duty to keep themselves well turns on a reciprocal relationship with the welfare state. Not only do we have a duty to make financial contributions to the system, but there is an additional duty for everybody to

refrain from putting avoidable strain on the system. Smoking and drinking to excess, eating a diet high in salt and saturated fat, and failing to exercise regularly all constitute violations of the duty we have to preserve the public purse. The request for costly treatment alternatives that offer no additional benefit over and above those that are cheaper and already in existence would be considered unjustifiable because it would constitute avoidable strain.

Further examination of this principle, however, reveals that it is far from robust, because it assumes that there is no such thing as random adversity and that health is under the direct control of the individual. The idea would be that, the harder we try, the better our health will be. Clearly, this is simply not sustainable in terms of disease aetiology. Even when there appears to be a strong correlation between behaviour and ill health, in order to say people are actually responsible for their difficulties, you have to be able to show beyond reasonable doubt that their own chosen behaviour caused the problem, and that they could have reasonably foreseen that the illness from which they now suffer would, by necessity, follow such behaviour.

For the sake of argument, let us suppose that all ill health is a function of reckless behaviour. To demonstrate fairness in distributing resources in this way, education programmes explaining the association between behaviour and disease would have to be universally accessible and consumers of health care would have to be committed to the lifestyle imperatives believed to promote the highest level of health.

Even so, effort would be very difficult to measure and evaluate, and what would happen to those who tried extremely hard but nevertheless succumbed to serious illness that was exceedingly costly to treat?

Benefit should be allocated in terms of the societal contributions of individuals

This material principle is often exposed by the popular example of who gets the last bed in intensive care. Should it be the hard working father of three or the alcoholic beggar who lives on the street? This issue of whether societal contribution warrants greater allocation of health care resource requires health care providers to grade the needs of competing groups. If contribution to society is to be the guiding principle, then those who have lived longest are likely to receive the most. In contrast, the concept of quality

17

adjusted life years (QALYs) would deny elderly people a favourable share because it is inclined towards the young and able-bodied, distributing benefit in accordance with *current* or *potential* contributions as opposed to previous contributions. Most vulnerable under such a system are those who have not, cannot, and never will make any contribution to society by virtue of forces far outside their own control. In this group we would include those born with physical or mental disability and those youngsters who develop disabilities in childhood or adolescence.

An ethical framework for prescribing

In financially constrained contexts, GPs—like all other health professionals—have a duty to ensure that the best value for money is obtained in order to maximise health care provision. This prescribing framework acknowledges that the local community assists in the delivery of its own health care through the collection of taxes. These funds are held in trust and therefore prescribers have a duty—not merely a responsibility—to provide the most effective treatments and therapies at the cheapest cost. The main advantage of an ethical framework for prescribing is that it causes the prescriber to think through the cost effectiveness as well as the clinical effectiveness questions critically, so it allows for some consistency in decision making. In addition, its structure calls for a regard for the evidence base which is not merely a clinical consideration, but first and foremost an ethical one. The reader is now referred to the framework (Fig 2.1) and, in the next section, the questions to be answered in chronological order are elaborated upon. The first working example assumes that the GP has been confronted by a patient who is requesting the beclomethasone dry powder delivery system as opposed to a standard metered dose inhaler (MDI) for the treatment of her asthma. The first is an expensive delivery system that has only ever been shown to have equivalent therapeutic effect to standard MDIs, the second being half the cost.[9] In the case of this particular patient, considerations about whether she can coordinate the use of the cheaper inhaler do not apply. It will be shown that the clinician, in appealing to the ethical framework, will clearly be able to justify her decision not to comply with this request based only on the answers to the first two questions.

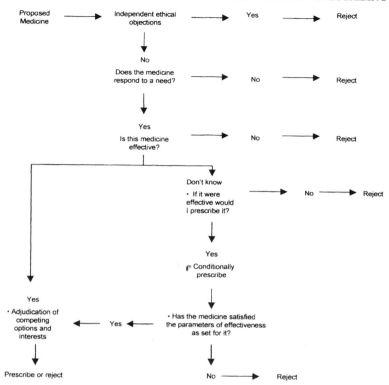

Figure 2.1   An ethical decision making model for prescribing medicines
Source: Kate Tunna, Department of General Practice, Birmingham University

Question 1: Is there an independent ethical objection to the proposed treatment?

In other words is there anything inherently wrong with the medicine that is being asked for? This question recognises that it is possible for treatments and therapies to be inherently wrong despite having potentially good effects. An example would be the Human Fertilisation and Embryology Authority's decision, following public consultation, not to permit the harvesting of ova from aborted fetuses for use in the treatment of infertility. Another example that may have more relevance to general practice would be treatment with hormone replacement therapy in which the source of oestrogen would be the urine of pregnant mares. There are some very pressing animal welfare concerns in the synthesis of

19

these hormones, including tethering of animals for excessive periods of time, subjecting horses to repeated pregnancies, and premature separation of mares and foals.

In short, it is suggested that an inherently unethical treatment would evidence one or more of the following characteristics:

- It would be derived unethically.
- It would be unnecessarily costly.
- It would offer little chance of beneficial outcome.
- It is associated with unethical clinical trials.
- The treatment itself may have a deleterious effect on the patient's dignity, an example of which would be that it prolongs the patient's suffering but provides no quantitative or qualitative benefit.

Obviously, it is not the job of GPs to act as guardians of morality; their attention should be directed at providing the best available treatment while at the same time ensuring the most prudent use of resources. Both doctors and patients may wish, however, to be mindful of the broader social and political issues, and discover from within the bounds of their own relationship whether any of these considerations render a particular therapy morally objectionable.

The more expensive delivery system could be rejected at this first stage in the decision tree because it is *unnecessarily* costly and therefore it would be intrinsically wrong to prescribe it. The published literature has shown that it offers no additional clinical benefit over and above what is currently considered best practice.

Question 2: Does this medicine respond to a need?

As it is impossible to give everyone everything they need, the job is to assess need in terms of severity and competing priority. The decision here calls for the balancing of harms and benefits, the overarching aim of course being to maximise benefit and minimise harm. The ethical principles of non-maleficence and beneficence force us to ask, first, whether the patient would actually be harmed if the expensive delivery system were not prescribed and, second, how much better off would she be if the particular treatment requested were prescribed. The doctor has to calculate the difference between the patient's asthma management now and what it might be like if this delivery system were prescribed. If it is the case that the patient's condition would improve with the

treatment she requests, then her need for that particular therapy would be accentuated. As will be explained more fully in Question 3, the doctor will have to assess the evidence in order to answer the question of relative effectiveness.

It is worth bearing in mind here how much drug advertising promulgates the belief that things would be so much better for the patient if the drug in question were prescribed. Assessment of the evidence provides a sturdy resistance to this kind of advertising which is undeniably persuasive. As it happens, research has shown that dry powder devices provide nothing more than what is currently considered best practice in terms of clinical effect. In the case of the asthma patient, there is clearly a need for inhaled corticosteroid therapy and it would be grossly unethical to fail to provide it. This mode of treatment is in existence, it works, and it relieves the signs and symptoms of a potentially life threatening disease, suffered by thousands of people in this country. To comply with the patient's request for a specific delivery device would not harm her directly—it would do the job—but it would not offer any additional clinical benefit to what is already available. Importantly, however, the cost of this medicine could lead to the harm of others if, in prescribing it, they might be deprived of treatments that were equally badly needed. On this basis alone, the doctor cannot justify prescribing this delivery device for this patient.

Question 3: Is this medicine effective?

Rather more than being described as a *trend*, there is an ethical imperative to assess the effectiveness of proposed treatments and therapies. Providing ineffective therapy is unjust in at least two ways. First, those who receive treatment of dubious or unproven value are denied the benefits of better treatments should they exist and, second, people will be denied access to effective services because others are receiving ineffective services that waste resources. Clinicians have an ethical responsibility to avail themselves of the best published literature and to develop their capacity to appraise it critically and then apply it. Viewed in this light, evidence based practice is every bit an ethical as it is a clinical imperative.

It would be wrong to say that the delivery system was ineffective as a treatment for asthma, so the best answer to Question 3 would be "yes". The route the doctor would then have to follow on the ethical decision making framework would take her to "adjudication

between competing therapies". In the present example, in view of the fact that the delivery system is no *more* effective than what is currently the best available alternative, it would be wrong to prescribe it, because it would place an unnecessary drain on resources. Reasoning her way through the framework, the doctor has ample justification to reject the patient's request on defensible ethical grounds.

Conditional prescribing

Now let us suppose that the answer to Question 3, "Is this therapy effective?" was "don't know". For this example, let us suppose the doctor has been asked to prescribe a topical non-steroidal gel for the treatment of arthritis. She has reviewed the evidence and found it to be equivocal—some sources are positive, others are not. One of the doctor's colleagues claims to have had good results with the gel and believes it is worth a try, at least. In this situation she decides that she will prescribe on a conditional basis. In other words she will conduct a micro trial of this particular treatment for this particular patient's condition. She will do this only after she has sought the valid consent of the patient, fully explaining the experimental nature of the undertaking. Both must agree to withdrawal of treatment if, after an appropriate trial period has elapsed, the desired outcomes—also agreed upon by doctor and patient—have not been reached.

Echoing Heather Draper's statement with regard to conditional purchasing, conditional prescribing would allow the doctor, "some escape from the twofold paralysis which can result from a commitment to effectiveness".[1] For one thing, effectiveness data may not be available in every case. In the case of new medicines it may be equivocal or contradictory, or the medicine in question is to be prescribed for indications outside its licensed use. Second, evidence may attest to the benefit of a new, improved preparation over and above what is currently available, but the cost is also far greater. Setting effectiveness criteria and the trial period time frame, again with a full understanding provided for the patient, the doctor will attempt treatment with the existing, less expensive treatment, progressing to the more expensive, newer alternative if the outcomes as set are not reached. No doubt there will be clinical emergencies that appear to necessitate prescribing the newer, more costly drug in the first instance, but generally speaking the least costly, best

available therapy should be implemented first. As with any clinical trial, the principal investigator, in this case the GP, must monitor the patient and gather relevant data as the trial is progressing and carefully record the results. The results of the conditional prescribing exercise lead to the next issue in the framework, namely deciding whether or not the parameters of effectiveness set for the treatment have been satisfied.

Conditional prescribing has the potential to promote both the clinician's autonomy and the best interests of the patient. In the long term, on the basis of replicated micro trials, a patient group may be serviced more effectively and therefore more justly, even in the absence of empirical norms. But the success and potential benefits of conditional prescribing demand that clinicians act responsibly in the face of the existing evidence. Conditional prescribing is not a means through which doctors can evade the sometimes burdensome task of critically appraising the literature. Tempting though it may be amidst the ever increasing pressures of general practice, doctors should be aware of the empirically derived measure of efficacy (or lack of it) that their proposed treatment carries. For reasons already discussed, this is integral to their clinical and ethical obligation to patients.

Finally, we will assume that the medicine has satisfied the measures of effectiveness set for it on the basis of negotiation between doctor and patient. To recap, the reasoning process entered into through the ethical framework has revealed that, for the medicine in question, there are no intrinsic ethical objections and it does respond to a need. Its effectiveness is uncertain, however, and so it has been prescribed on condition that it meets the measures of effectiveness set for it. The last hurdle in prescribing has to do with continuing to provide this treatment over the long term. If the doctor is willing to undertake conditional purchase, then to be fair he or she must allow a reasonable trial period to elapse before deciding whether or not the effectiveness criteria have been reached. Depending upon the patient's condition and the proposed treatment, a reasonable trial period could range from hours to months.

Having reached the final cross roads of decision making means that grounds to reject prescribing the treatment in question have not yet been found. One final question remains and as the doctor faces the patient in the surgery this may, psychologically, be the most difficult. The competition for resources may be so

23

great that the decision about who will get what they want and who will not can seem utterly impossible. The playing field is uneven. Different health authorities will have made different decisions about what is to be made available to patients. The patient's post code can have as much to do with the services and treatments that are available to them as can the particular ailment that they have.

Until quite recently, GPs were able to avoid the task of priority setting in relation to their own patient populations but the era of fundholding, with its responsibility for the local disbursement of a finite budget, meant that they had to become significant players in these matters of health care politics. Fundholding was essentially a cost saving exercise and the promise that it held has been clouded by the ever shrinking purchasing capacity of every single pound. The tension between their roles as both purchaser and provider may well be greatest for fundholders as they arrive at this final point in the model—adjudicating between the competing demands and needs of their patients. The principles of health care delivery described by Goodwin[8] as effectiveness, efficiency, equity, and humanity apply at every level. The difficulty in upholding these principles stems from the problem of limited resource which means that not all needs can be met. Sometimes patient and indeed clinician autonomy will have to be sacrificed in the service of more pressing demands and harm may occur to a patient as a result. Provided that the process of adjudication was just, it cannot be claimed that the doctor has wronged the patient. GPs, like all others involved in health care delivery, cannot do the impossible; however, they must be able to show that they did their absolute best to minimise harm and maximise good in the financial circumstances within which they were operating.

How doctors in general practice should adjudicate between competing needs is beyond the scope of this chapter, because it will depend to such a large extent on individual practice and patient population variables. McKeown's[10] warning against, "all those who claim to have the right answers to offer" (page 27) is reassuring to all of us who contemplate this kind of decision making with a heavy heart, sympathetic to the GPs, yet thankful that it is not our responsibility. Considerations such as urgency, severity, age, potential to benefit, and responsibility for health as discussed in this chapter may have proportional relevance in any given situation. The belief is that an ethical reasoning process, such as that offered

by this prescribing framework, will help doctors to reach justifiable decisions. At the very least its conscientious use can free the practitioner from any accusation by hospital colleagues, patients, or the industry of inequitable treatment.

1 Draper H, Tunna K. *Ethics and values for commissioners. A report by the Yorkshire Collaborating Centre for Health Services Research.* Leeds: Nuffield Institute for Health, 1996.
2 Pellegrino ED, Thomasma DC. *A philosophical basis of medical practice: towards a philosophy and ethic of the healing professions.* Oxford: Oxford University Press, 1981.
3 Veatch R. *Case studies in medical ethics.* Boston, MA: Harvard University Press, 1977.
4 Beauchamp T, Childress J. *Principles of biomedical ethics.* Oxford: Oxford University Press, 1994.
5 Gillon R. Defending the "four principles approach" to biomedical ethics. *J Med Ethics* 1995;**21**:323–4.
6 Holm S. Not just autonomy: the principles of American biomedical ethics. *J Med Ethics* 1995;**21**:332–8.
7 Rawls J. *A theory of justice.* London: Oxford University Press, 1972.
8 Goodwin S. Commissioning for health. *Health Visitor* 1995;**68**:16–18.
9 Anon. Delivery systems for inhaled asthma therapy. *Drug Therapy Persp* 1997;**9**:8–9.
10 McKeown K, Whitelaw S, Hambleton D, Green F. Setting priorities: science, art or politics. In: *Setting priorities in health care* (Malek M, ed.). Chichester: John Wiley, 1994.

3 A primary care perspective on medicines management

COLIN BRADLEY

Objectives

- To highlight patterns and trends in UK primary care prescribing and make some limited international comparisons.
- To discuss the scope for altering prescribing patterns based on research on spontaneous changes and changes brought about by specific policy initiatives.
- To describe and highlight the problems associated with repeat prescribing systems.
- To suggest an agenda for practices to reform their prescribing policies.
- To draw attention to the range of additional support mechanisms.

The activities of primary care physicians, that is, general practitioners in the UK context, have a major influence on medicines management. About 80% of all prescriptions written are written in primary care and the drugs dispensed against these prescriptions cost over £4000 million per annum in 1995–96.[1] This is over 12% of the whole NHS budget and is more than 50% of the entire cost of providing family practitioner services.[2] The prescribing patterns of UK general practitioners are scrutinised intensively by various agencies including their contracting health authority, the Department of Health, and researchers. This scrutiny has been greatly facilitated by the computerisation of the system for the reimbursement of pharmacists which can now also produce detailed information on prescribing habits. This electronic database

is used to generate several different forms of written feedback to each prescriber and is described in chapter 6.

Trends and patterns in primary care prescribing

These statistics show that the total quantity of drugs is rising year on year, as is their total cost. This is occurring in spite of a fairly static population growth. The possible reasons for this are discussed in chapter 4. Within this overall pattern of rising costs and volume of drugs used, major differences in drug usage between regions, between practices, and between individual prescribers have been observed. There have been many attempts to account for these variations, in terms of the measurable parameters and of what might reasonably be expected to drive drug use. The literature is confusing and sometimes even contradictory, but it seems that prescribing patterns in practices are certainly related to the numbers of patients on the list and their age–sex mix. Older patients and female patients generally require more medicines and, hence, incur greater drugs expenditure. One would expect prescribing volume and, hence, cost to be related to morbidity but obtaining evidence of this is difficult. This is, in part, because of the difficulties of obtaining good morbidity data from general practice, but may also be because the effects of morbidity on prescribing patterns are being confounded by the idiosyncrasies of individual prescribers. There are some data, however, which do indicate that morbidity, and various proxies for morbidity (such as days of sickness absence), are related to prescribing costs and volumes. A link between material deprivation and morbidity has been well established but this is not well borne out in prescribing patterns. Studies seeking to link prescribing patterns to measures of deprivation have not shown any consistent association, as might have been expected, although some markers of deprivation, such as unemployment levels, have been found to be associated with higher prescribing levels.

Studies of the prescribing patterns of individual doctors show that there is great variation between doctors even when facing apparently similar patient populations. McGavock, in a study of high and low cost prescribers in Belfast, showed that, although high cost practices did appear to have higher morbidity rates, they also prescribed more symptomatic remedies and tended to issue prescriptions for larger quantities of medicines.[3] Similarly, the

27

Audit Commission compared the prescribing of 54 practices, whose prescribing they judged to be close to optimal, with the national patterns.[4] Five main ways in which patterns seemed to deviate from this standard were noted, namely:

- Underprescribing of more expensive drugs with greater clinical impact (for example, inhaled corticosteroids in asthma).
- Prescribing drugs of limited clinical value (for example, vasodilators).
- Prescribing of drugs with specific indications more frequently than would be predicted from the prevalence of the indications.
- Prescribing drugs for which there was an equally effective but cheaper (often generic) alternative.
- Prescribing of *premium price* preparations more often than seems justified by their added cost.

The Audit Commission estimated that, if all practices were to follow the pattern they observed in their study practices, a saving of £425 million annually could be made on the drugs bill for England and Wales.

International comparisons

However fraught with difficulties studies of prescribing patterns within the UK are, with its national system for health care provision and reasonably comprehensive and reliable prescribing data, it is nothing compared with the difficulties of making international comparisons of patterns of drug use. When such international comparisons are made, what is most striking is how different countries, even those sharing a broadly similar medical culture, are from each other. Thus, in one study, the French were found to consume an average of 38 prescription items per annum, the Italians 20, the Germans 12, the British 7.6, and the Dutch 6.9. Garattini and Garattini,[5] in another study, found that, of the 50 most commonly sold products in Italy, France, Germany, and the UK, only seven were common to all four countries. In addition to differences in cultures of medicines use, differences in morbidity patterns and use of morbidity labels, differences in demographic patterns, and differences in Government regulatory policies and practices mean that drawing any sensible conclusions from different patterns of drug use is virtually impossible. Broadly speaking, however, it seems that the UK pattern is of a relatively low rate of

usage which is more restricted than prescribing in many other countries.

Changing prescribing patterns

Given the large sums involved and the marked variations observed, many parties are interested in how prescribing patterns change and what sorts of influences lead to changes in prescribing. Taylor and Bond,[6] in a study of the initial prescribing of a drug new to a doctor's repertoire, found that prescribing of a drug for the first time occurred in only 5.4% of initial prescriptions. When it did occur, the two principal influences tended to be pharmaceutical company marketing, especially via company representatives and recommendations from consultant specialist colleagues. The last tended to be influential across a wider range of treatments, whereas company representatives were a prominent influence mainly for prescribing of remedies confined to general practice use, particularly antibiotics and analgesics. They also found that new drugs did not simply replace older drugs that had become obsolete, but tended to be added to the repertoire with older drugs probably fading from use more slowly. This confirmed earlier research which showed drug acquisition and drug relinquishment to be distinct processes under different influences. Armstrong,[7] in a qualitative study of GPs' reasons for changing their prescribing, found that change seemed to be brought about by one of three types of change process:

- Change occurred as a result of an accumulation of evidence in favour of the change.
- A single dramatic event seemed to bring about the change, such as the occurrence of an adverse drug reaction.
- Changes seemed to occur because the doctor was ready to change for other reasons.

Thus, a new drug may have been launched that seemed to fulfil a need of which the doctor was already aware. Deliberate attempts to alter the prescribing behaviour of doctors have relied on these and many other observations indicating that doctors' prescribing is amenable to change through educational processes. This is also the philosophical basis that supports education outreach programmes such as those described in chapter 10.

Change can, however, be brought about, often much more dramatically, by changes in regulations and policies governing prescribing. Thus, for example, the blacklisting in 1985 of several groups of drugs, and so prohibiting their prescription on the NHS, led to a virtual cessation of prescribing of the drugs in question. Such crude attempts to alter prescribing can, however, have unpredictable effects. Thus, the 1985 limited list led to some classes of drugs, such as cough mixtures, being virtually eradicated, whereas in others, such as antacids, the banned products were substituted with other products that could, in some cases, be more expensive.[8] Similarly, prescription charges levied on patients do seem to reduce demand for medicines, but the effect seems to be short lived and there is some evidence that patients at the borderline of eligibility may be failing to receive necessary medicines. The GP fundholding scheme is a more subtle alteration to the prescribing milieu, which gives GPs more discretion but still introduces a financial rigour perceived to have been absent heretofore. The evidence discussed in chapter 6 suggests that fundholding does, indeed, lead to some cost containment of prescribing expenditure without any apparent disadvantages to patients, although these effects seem to be less for later waves of fundholding and there is now some suspicion that early gains in cost containment are not sustained over time. Incentive schemes for non-fundholders have started to demonstrate that similar changes can be brought about by other forms of financial incentive to limit prescribing expenditure. It has been found that, in both these schemes, doctors' drug selection decisions are altered more readily than decisions about whether or not to issue a prescription.

Repeat prescribing

Repeat prescribing systems have evolved in UK general practice to deal with the need for patients to have long term medications re-prescribed without the need to see the doctor on each and every occasion. The theoretical benefits are that the patient does not have to get a doctor's appointment or have to wait to see the doctor, and the doctor's time is not taken up with patients for whom little or nothing has to be done. Such systems are supposed to have built into them times for regular review and, because these are less frequent, the doctor will feel more obliged to check everything that needs to be monitored and so the patient gets

less frequent but more thorough check ups. Changes in medical practice, with increasing proportions of older people with chronic degenerative conditions now making up the bulk of primary medical care, have led to repeat prescribing becoming more prevalent. The latest estimates suggest that somewhere between two thirds and three quarters of all items are now issued on repeat prescription.[9]

Zermansky[10] has described the three components of repeat prescribing systems:

- A production component which is how requests are handled administratively and the actual prescription is produced for evaluation and signing by the doctor and transmission back to the patient (or his or her representative).
- A management component which ensures that the patient who requests a prescription is actually entitled to one and ensures that patients are receiving prescriptions at the appropriate time, that is, not too soon and not too late.
- A clinical component in which the doctor determines that the patient is on the appropriate medication(s), has sufficient information about his or her medication and its further supply, and is being seen at the appropriate intervals for monitoring of the relevant parameters.

In his study of repeat prescribing in 50 practices in Leeds, Zermansky identified multiple deficiencies at all levels of the systems he studied. He suggests, in particular, that more time needs to be given to clinical review and questions whether this could be delegated to pharmacists or, subject to suitable training, nurses.

A primary care prescribing agenda

The concerns raised above on the variability of prescribing from doctor to doctor and practice to practice and the ever increasing drugs bill mean that the pressure for reform in general practice prescribing is unlikely to abate in the foreseeable future. Educational efforts and legislative pressures will continue to be applied to try to bring all general practice prescribing up to the standard of what is perceived to be the best. In this climate, practices will need to examine their prescribing and ensure that it can be fully justified on both clinical and economic grounds. This should be done systematically and policies set in place so that

important prescribing decisions can be made with maximum information and group consensus, rather than always being made under pressure in the heat of consultations. To this end we should examine:

- The need for prescriptions in some instances.
- The evidence base supporting prescribing.
- The scope for maximising the cost effectiveness of prescribing.
- The operation of any repeat prescribing system.

The need for prescriptions

There are relatively few instances in which the need for a medication is absolute rather than relative. Exceptions are replacement therapies such as insulin for type 1 diabetes mellitus. In very many instances of both acute and chronic conditions seen in general practice, the only treatment available is one that merely relieves symptoms but does not alter the course of the illness. All symptomatic treatment is potentially discretionary, and decisions to prescribe symptomatic remedies and how frequently relate more to attitudes to medicines use in general, than to a scientific understanding of drugs and their effects. Patients' attitudes are also an influence and different patients with similar symptoms will vary in the extent to which they see treatment as either necessary or desirable.

Research suggests that doctors are often unaware of the patient's view and that it is the doctor's attitude that dictates whether or not a prescription is issued. On the other hand, there is also some evidence (see chapter 6) that there are occasions on which the doctor does not believe the medicine to be justified, but it is issued anyway because of the perceived wishes of the patient. This applies not just to medicines that might be deemed symptomatic, but may apply to medicines with specific uses that may not be justified for the particular patient. It seems that there is a communication gap between doctors and their patients about the necessity for some prescriptions and, where the treatment is purely symptomatic, the patient's and doctor's views may be considered equally valid. It should be possible to resolve such differences in belief and perspective by dialogue although this may require negotiation skills, especially on the part of the doctor.

The evidence base supporting prescribing

Although it is true to say that all drugs must now be subjected to rigorous clinical trials before being marketed, this is not to say that all prescribing is in fact evidence based. The application of evidence to clinical medicine requires that doctors look at the relevance and the quality of the evidence before applying it to their practice. To this end, they need to develop the skills and expertise for assessing original and derived evidence, to determine whether it is of sufficient quality and relevance for application to any particular practice situation. The ways of assessing the evidence are discussed in chapter 5. In considering whether to adopt a therapy in primary care, however, there are some common pitfalls in the evidence that need to be avoided. It is also necessary to look at how similar patients in the trial are to your own patients. Thus results of trials conducted in a specialised setting on a highly selected population will not automatically be transferable to a general practice population. Trials are usually conducted on patients who are fairly ill with a well defined diagnosis. Results from such a trial are not transferable to patients less dramatically afflicted or in whom the diagnosis is more presumptive.

Any trial should compare new therapy with current best treatment and not just placebo. Placebo controls are demanded by regulatory authorities whose duty it is to establish efficacy of the drug, but for clinicians it is comparative efficacy that is at issue and so a placebo control is only appropriate for conditions for which there is currently no treatment. Trial end points should also relate to patient outcome—did the patients live or die, get worse, better, or stay the same? Proxy end points, such as laboratory markers of disease or even pain scores and the like, are less satisfactory than true clinical end points such as death or disability. Finally, the design of the trial is not the only concern. It is necessary to look at how it was carried out and at such matters as how results were analysed. For instance, analysis should be on an intention to treat basis, that is, with dropouts included in the arm to which they were randomised rather than omitted from analysis.

Maximising cost effectiveness of prescribing

The first step in this is often to eliminate prescribing that is needlessly expensive. The most obvious way to do this is by

prescribing generically.[11] The evidence suggests that many GPs are already doing this; generic prescribing rates have been rising steadily for almost a decade, although some doctors have residual concerns about comprehensive generic prescribing. Indeed, there are some areas of prescribing in which generic substitution is not necessarily appropriate, in particular, for drugs with a narrow therapeutic index. Examples of such drugs would include anticonvulsants, such as carbamazepine and phenytoin, and cyclosporin and lithium.

Generic prescribing of modified release formulations of drugs is also usually undesirable; there are many instances in which a modified release formulation, although available, is not necessary. The claimed advantage for many slow release preparations is that they aid compliance, but the difference in compliance between once daily and twice daily dosing is often negligible. There are many other areas where drugs in current use could be substituted by different but cheaper ones. The clinical benefits may be identical and the claimed advantages for the more expensive products may be irrelevant or may not apply to the particular patient being treated. As an example, the advantages claimed for isosorbide mononitrate that it is subject to less first pass metabolism and is better absorbed are simply not relevant for most patients most of the time. An even more contentious area is that which the Audit Commission called *premium price preparations*. These are preparations that are considerably more costly than the products for which they are offered as substitutes. Although these preparations may have advantages over existing products, the advantage is not sufficient to justify the price premium—certainly not for all relevant patients. An example of this is the newer, more sophisticated delivery systems for asthma drugs. Although these are often more convenient for patients, the therapeutic benefit is often only marginal whereas the cost differential is substantial.

Maximising cost effectiveness, however, does not always mean prescribing more cheaply. It may, on occasion, even involve prescribing a more expensive preparation. An example of this, cited by the Audit Commission, is the use of inhaled corticosteroids in the treatment of asthma in preference to inhaled bronchodilators. Unfortunately, determining the most cost effective treatment is often not that straightforward. Ideally, cost effectiveness should be determined on the basis of an appropriate health economic evaluation (see chapter 7) but, although there is clinical trial evidence to support the use of most drugs, economic evaluations

are much rarer. Furthermore, many of the economic evaluations available are somewhat suspect, having been funded by the pharmaceutical industry to make a case for an expensive therapy the clinical justification for which may be rather weak. There are now standards for the appraisal of economic evaluations similar to those available for clinical trials, but few GPs have a sufficient understanding of basic health economics to be able to apply them. This is likely to become an area for development in the future of primary care prescribing.

The operation of repeat prescribing systems

As mentioned above, Zermansky[10] has highlighted the problems in this area and in particular insufficient clinical control being exerted by doctors. Part of the problem may be that repeat prescribing is not set up very flexibly and so it fails to deal efficiently with the differing needs of patients. Some may be being reviewed more often than is strictly necessary, with the result that the review process becomes empty and ritualised. Other patients, however, go for too long between reviews and their medicine taking becomes increasingly chaotic due to lack of sufficient guidance. What is needed is a greater distinction to be drawn between chronic stable conditions and more volatile situations, and between medicines that are disease modifying (and, hence, virtually essential) and drugs that are more symptom controlling (and, hence, more optional). For chronic stable conditions in which a disease modifying drug is used, after a period of close monitoring for adverse reactions and stabilisation, review intervals can be lengthened to match the requirements of monitoring of either the disease or its treatment. For many such situations there are now consensus based, and increasingly evidence based, guidelines to inform repeat prescribing policy. For less stable situations, or where drugs are being used on an *as required* basis, a longer period may be required to determine the pattern of need and use of drugs. Once the usual levels of drug use have been determined, review intervals can be lengthened to match any needs to monitor disease or drug. Provision may still need to be made for a speedy route back into closer review if the situation destabilises. The implementation of such a policy would lead to more variable patterns of review of people on long term medications, instead of the current virtually standard intervals of one, two, three, and six months.

Support systems for GP prescribing

Given the pressures on GPs in the prescribing arena and, in particular, the need to make changes one might ask how GPs could go about implementing the new approach and who might help them in this.[12] The first step is to try to shift the arena for prescribing decisions from the heat of the consultation to other situations where the benefits of various treatments might be considered in greater detail. The reality of general practice is that many prescribing decisions are made recurrently. The opportunity to consider the decision in advance of the encounter with the patient should make it easier for the doctor to adhere to principles of rational prescribing. What is needed is for GPs to meet together and consider in more detail, under conditions of less pressure, their common prescribing decisions. This will involve detailed consideration of the various drugs and medicinal preparations available to them. Information will be needed on the preparations available and the trial evidence supporting their use in various situations. Although it is possible for GPs to obtain this information for themselves, it is difficult and laborious. Pharmacists can be very helpful in this regard, particularly if they have been trained in the specialist area of *drug information.*[13] A number of practices have employed pharmacists in such an information and advisory role and have generally been pleased with the results. Another potential source of assistance with such endeavours is the professional advisers at health authorities.

Although, at first, professional advisers were mostly doctors who had a very wide brief which in practice precluded such detailed work with individual practices, there are now more pharmacists, some of whom are specifically deployed to help with practice initiatives. If demand from practices were to rise, I have little doubt that the supply of such pharmaceutical support would be increased to meet it. Finally, a much underutilised resource in this regard is the community pharmacist. An increasing proportion of community pharmacists will have been through a training that will have familiarised them with both the pharmacological and the therapeutic aspects of most modern drugs. From a training point of view they are well equipped to offer information and to support decision making, especially in the selection of drugs. Their work situation and their obligation to be present when prescriptions are dispensed limit their capacity to come to practices to offer advice

and support. With more flexible arrangements for the delivery of primary care still being considered, however, it seems probable that this capacity of community pharmacists may yet be properly exploited.

Another primary care resource that is coming into the prescribing arena is that of the practice nurse. Nurse prescribing was introduced in 1994 on a fairly limited basis. Certain nurses with district nursing or health visitor qualifications in eight demonstration sites were allowed, after some additional training, to prescribe from a limited formulary. Since then the scheme has been expanded to encompass all health districts and the formulary has been expanded slightly, including the introduction to the formulary of six preparations previously only prescribable by doctors. Initial evaluation of nurse prescribing found it to be favourably received by doctors, nurses, and patients, and some of the anticipated problems did not materialise. It is early days, however, and although nurse prescribing is set to expand geographically, it may be some time before its scope is expanded to a level that would negate the need for GPs to sign or countersign prescriptions. This fails to recognise the considerable expansion of nurses into a very active involvement in chronic disease management, including effectively making therapeutic decisions. A more fruitful way forward may be for collaboration between nurses and pharmacists in chronic disease management and its drug treatment, which may allow the doctor to disengage safely from routine care in reasonably stable cases. This may be facilitated under new arrangements being developed in primary care, which allow practices to employ or contract pharmacists more directly as part of a practice team.

Conclusion

Medicines use in primary care is too important an issue both clinically and economically to be allowed to elude management. Although by international comparisons medicines management in the UK may be seen to be reasonably tight, the large variations between regions, practices, and prescribers which defy rational explanation suggest that there is still scope for improvement. Studies of spontaneous changes in prescribing practice have encouraged educational attempts to persuade doctors to alter their prescribing with the goal of maximising cost effectiveness. It is suggested here that practices need to take this on board and begin

to set a prescribing agenda which should address the initial need for any medicine, the evidence base supporting any given medicines use, the economics of prescribing, and the operation of the repeat prescribing system. Efforts to undertake these reforms need support from the health authorities and particularly their professional prescribing advisers, but practices themselves may seek support from other sources, particularly pharmacists and nurses.

Key points

- There are wide variations in prescribing in primary care that cannot be fully accounted for by demography or morbidity patterns.
- Prescribing patterns of primary care physicians are amenable to change by educational processes and by policy initiatives. The effects of the second tend to be more dramatic but less predictable.
- Repeat prescribing is an important feature of UK primary care which seems at the moment to be poorly managed.
- Practices should set a prescribing agenda that addresses the need to prescribe in the first place, the evidence base supporting prescribing, the maximisation of cost effectiveness and the tighter regulation of repeat prescribing.
- There are now more support mechanisms to aid GPs in these responsibilities, including pharmacists and, possibly, nurses.

1 Government Statistical Service. *Statistics of prescriptions dispensed in the Family Practitioner Services Authorities: England 1985–1995*. London: Department of Health, 1996.
2 Prescription Pricing Authority. *Annual Report*. Newcastle upon Tyne: Prescription Pricing Authority, 1996.
3 McGavock H. Some patterns of prescribing by urban general practitioners. *BMJ* 1988;**296**:900–2.
4 Audit Commission. *A prescription for improvement: towards more rational prescribing in general practice*. London: HMSO, 1994.
5 Garattini S, Garattini L. Pharmaceutical prescriptions in four European countries. *Lancet* 1993;**342**:1191–2.
6 Taylor R, Bond C. Change in the established prescribing habits of general practitioners: an analysis of initial prescriptions in general practice. *Br J Gen Pract* 1991;**41**:244–8.
7 Armstrong D. A study of general practitioners' reasons for changing their prescribing behaviour. *BMJ* 1996;**312**:949–52.

8 Griffin J, Griffin D. The economic implications of therapeutic conservatism. *J R Coll Physicians Lond* 1993;**27**:121–6.
9 Harris CM, Dajdar R. The scale of repeat prescribing. *Br J Gen Pract* 1996; **46**:649–53.
10 Zermansky A. Who controls repeats? *Br J Gen Pract* 1996;**46**:643–7.
11 Mucklow J. Generic prescribing. *Prescribers J* 1997;**37**:133–7.
12 Hobbs F, Bradley C. *Prescribing in primary care*. Oxford: Oxford University Press, 1998.
13 Bradley C, Taylor R, Blenkinsopp A. Developing prescribing in primary care. *BMJ* 1997;**314**:744–7.

4 Rising expenditure on medicines—reasons and responses

RHONA PANTON, ALAN EARL-SLATER,
ELENA GRANT

Objectives

- To review the rise in expenditure on medicines.
- To identify and examine Government initiatives on their use.
- To review purchasers' responses.
- To outline the range of policies on pharmaceutical expenditure worldwide.
- To consider the response of the pharmaceutical industry to these policies.

The change in the NHS drugs bill

Factors driving the drugs bill upwards have been extensively reviewed.[1] Four key drivers of cost are: demographic change, new drugs and delivery systems, Government policy, and increasing awareness and expectation of patients and health care professionals. Drug expenditure in 1980–96 is shown in Fig 4.1 using the net ingredient cost of drugs.[2] The change in expenditure is shown in Fig 4.2 using the net ingredient cost (NIC, the cost of the drug) adjusted for inflation (by the Government's gross domestic product or GDP at factor cost and using 1996 prices as a base).

Between 1980 and 1996 the NHS drugs bill increased by 126% in real terms and the rate of rise was markedly increased from

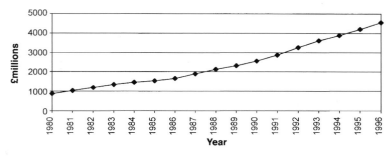

Figure 4.1   The National Health Service drugs bill 1980–1996 United Kingdom
Source: Compendium of Health Statistics 10th Edition. London: Office of
Health Economics.

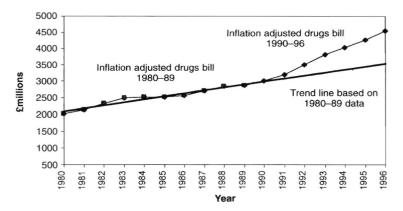

Figure 4.2   The inflation adjusted drugs bill 1980–96 United Kingdom
Source: Keele University prescribing analysis.
Note: 1996 prices are used as a base.

1989. If the trend of the 1980s had continued, the 1996 drugs bill
would be 27% lower.

Demographic trends

In 1960, 16.4 million people in the UK were under 15 years of
age (31%) and 6.3 million were over 65 years of age (12%). In
1996 the numbers were 15.4 million (26%) and 10.2 million (17%)
respectively.[3]

In 1996, an average elderly person in England received 22
prescription items (up from 12.2 in 1978), with children receiving

41

five prescriptions per year (up from 3.4 in 1978). Over all age groups the average number of prescription items dispensed was eight per person per year (up from 6.6 in 1978) (Fig 4.3)[2]

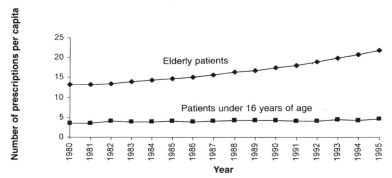

Figure 4.3 Prescription items dispensed by age group
Source: Compendium of Health Statistics 10th Edition. London: Office of Health Economics.

Elderly people receive almost three times as many prescriptions as the average younger person and the rate of rise is greatest in this age group. As they are also exempt prescription charges, any rise in the elderly population inevitably means a rise in the drugs bill.[1]

Obviously life for elderly people is much better than it was 50 years ago. Most of the medicines on which modern treatment relies so heavily were not even thought of. All but a handful of the antimicrobial drugs used routinely to treat infection were unavailable and infection was still a common cause of death. The treatment of cardiovascular diseases has been greatly improved by the introduction of β blockers, calcium antagonists, and angiotensin converting enzyme (ACE) inhibitors, not to mention thrombolytic therapy. The routine use of inhaled broncho-dilators and corticosteroids has changed asthma in most of those who have the condition from a disability into a nuisance. Non-steroidal anti-inflammatory agents have reduced the restriction of activity caused by painful musculoskeletal conditions, while painful dyspepsia can now invariably be relieved and sometimes cured without recourse to surgery. Finally, surgery itself has been facilitated and rendered much safer by modern anaesthetic agents. Those who rail about the inadequacies of health care in the 1990s should spare a thought for what it was like in the 1940s. By

Table 4.1 New indications for established drugs—some examples

Drug	Initial indication	New indication
Acyclovir	Herpes simplex, herpes zoster	Childhood and adolescent chickenpox
Alprostadil	Maintenance of patency of ductus arteriosus in neonates with congenital heart defects	Impotence
Cyclosporin	Prevention of organ and tissue transplant rejection and prophylaxis against graft versus host disease	Severe active rheumatoid arthritis Atopic dermatitis Severe psoriasis
Etidronate	Paget's disease, hypercalcaemia	Treatment of osteoporosis and prevention of postmenopausal osteoporosis
Fluticasone	Seasonal allergic rhinitis	Asthma
Interferon-α	Hairy cell leukaemia, recurrent or metastatic renal cell carcinoma, AIDS related Kaposi's sarcoma	Chronic active hepatitis B Chronic hepatitis C Malignant melanoma
Omeprazole	Zollinger–Ellison syndrome Oesophageal reflux disease Duodenal and benign gastric ulcer	*Helicobacter pylori* eradication
Methotrexate	Malignant disease	Rheumatoid arthritis Severe psoriasis

Source: West Midlands Drug Information Service.

comparison, we are rich beyond measure. New uses are also found for older drugs and Table 4.1 gives some examples. Some new drugs bring notable therapeutic advantages and the most important are shown in Table 4.2.

New drugs, delivery systems and new uses of older drugs

These all influence the NHS drugs bill. The main drivers are new drugs that have a large volume of sales, which are used for chronic or widespread conditions. Between 1989 and 1994 the change from older to newer more expensive products accounted for 55% of the total growth in the NHS drugs bill.[4] Tables 4.3 and 4.4 show the amount spent on some of these new drugs. Much

Table 4.2   Major therapeutic advances in the last 10 years

Therapeutic group	Indications
4-Quinolones	Bacterial infections
5HT$_3$ antagonists	Antiemetics for chemotherapy and radiotherapy and postoperative nausea and vomiting
Atypical antipsychotics	Schizophrenia
Erythropoietin	Anaemia associated with chronic renal failure and in adult cancer patients receiving platinum containing chemotherapy To increase yield of autologous blood in predonation programme Prevent anaemia of prematurity
Fibrinolytic drugs	Acute myocardial infarction Pulmonary embolism Deep vein thrombosis Thrombosed arteriovenous shunts Other thrombotic conditions
Growth hormone	Growth hormone deficiency in children and adults
Luteinising hormone releasing hormone (LHRH) analogues	Prostate cancer, advanced breast cancer, endometriosis and endometrial thinning, fertility
Nucleoside reverse transcriptase inhibitors (NRTIs)	HIV infection
Protease inhibitors	HIV infection
Proton pump inhibitors (PPIs)	Peptic ulcer disease, gastro-oesophageal reflux disease, acid related dyspepsia With antibiotics, *H. pylori* eradication
Pulmonary surfactants	Respiratory distress syndrome (RDS) in neonates
Recombinant human granulocyte–colony stimulating factor (rhG-CSF)	Reduction of chemotherapy induced neutropenia, thereby reducing the incidence of sepsis
Selective serotonin reuptake inhibitors (SSRIs)	Depression Obsessive compulsive disorder Panic disorder Bulimia nervosa
Statins	Hypercholesterolaemia Primary and secondary prevention of coronary heart disease
Vaccines	Immunisation against hepatitis A and B

Source: West Midlands Drug Information Service.

Table 4.3 Newer drugs contributing to the increase in expenditure

Old			New				
Drug group	Market leader (by spend)	Cost per defined daily dose[a]	Drug group	Market leader (by spend)	Cost per defined daily dose[a]	Percentage difference between the cost per defined daily dose of the older and newer drug	Annual expenditure for England on the new market leader (Jan–Dec 1996)
Tricyclic antidepressants	Lofepramine HCl tab 70mg	£0.26	Selective serotonin reuptake inhibitors	Fluoxetine HCl cap 20mg	£0.69	165	£63627600
H₂-receptor antagonists	Ranitidine HCl tab 150mg	£0.93	Proton pump inhibitors	Omeprazole cap e/c[b] 20mg	£1.27	37	£187290700
Non-steroidal anti-inflammatory drugs	Ibuprofen tab 400mg	£0.04	Non-steroidal anti-inflammatory drugs	Tenoxicam tab 20mg	£0.50	1150	£1473000
Penicillins	Amoxycillin cap 250mg	£0.15	4-Quinolones	Ciprofloxacin tab 250mg	£3.00	1900	£7792900
Angiotensin-converting enzyme inhibitors	Enalapril 20mg tab	£0.23	Angiotensin II receptor antagonists	Losartan tab 50mg	£0.62	170	£3772600
Calcium channel blockers	Nifedipine tab 20mg m/r[c]	£0.25	Calcium channel blockers	Amlodipine tab 5mg	£0.42	68	£36796600

[a] Defined daily dose (DDD)—the assumed average dose per day for a drug used on its main indication in adults as calculated by the World Health Organization. DDDs are used for cost comparison purposes only.
[b] e/c—enteric coated.
[c] m/r—modified release.
Source: based on West Midlands prescribing data provided by the Prescription Pricing Authority. Drug retail price data is taken from Drug Tariff or the Chemist & Druggist monthly price list for June 1997.

Table 4.4   Newer delivery systems contributing to the increase in expenditure

| Old market leader | | | New market leader | | | Percentage difference between the cost per defined daily dose of the older and the newer delivery system | Annual expenditure for England on the new delivery system (Jan–Dec 1996) |
Delivery system	Drug	Cost per defined daily dose[a]	Delivery system	Drug	Cost per defined daily dose[a]		
Metered dose inhaler	Salbutamol 100 µg	£0.07	Dry powder devices	Salbutamol 400 µg	£0.21	200	£6 293 500
Tablet	Oestradiol 1 mg	£0.17	Patch	Oestradiol 50 µg/24 hours	£0.27	200	£9 322 200
Tablet	Diclofenac Sodium tab e/c[b] 50 mg	£0.16	Sustained release tablet	Diclofenac Sodium m/r[c] tab 100 mg	£0.45	181	£20 681 800
Tablet	Ibuprofen tab 400 mg	£0.04	Sustained release tablet	Ibuprofen m/r[c] tab 800 mg	£0.31	675	£5 236 900

[a] Defined daily dose (DDD)—the assumed average dose per day for a drug used on its main indication in adults as calculated by the World Health Organization. DDDs are used for cost comparison purposes only.
[b] e/c—enteric coated.
[c] m/r—modified release.
Source: based on West Midlands prescribing data provided by the Prescription Pricing Authority. Drug retail price data is taken from Drug Tariff or the *Chemist & Druggist* monthly price list for June 1997.

higher media interest and concern among purchasers of health care is shown in making decisions about new drugs of high unit cost. Although the patient numbers may be smaller, the purchaser is required to review the evidence with awareness of the impact on other health services. An example is interferon-β for the treatment of certain patients with multiple sclerosis which costs £8000 per patient per year.

Government policies

The third influence on the NHS drugs bill is the collection of Government policies. This includes cash limits on hospital services, but not drug budgets in primary care, user charges, GP fundholding lists or products that cannot be reimbursed, changing prescription only status, advertising controls, the pharmaceutical and medical advisory structure for prescribing advice, and incentive schemes. Yet, at a population level, there is no robust evidence that this collection of policies complements rather than counteracts them. For example, encouragement of the pharmaceutical industry by promoting research and development conflicts with the policy to promote generic prescribing. There is clear conflict between cash limited hospitals and no clearly understood cash limit in primary care. The pharmaceutical industry has responded to this by offering large discounts to hospitals for drugs that will subsequently be used in primary care. These can be around 70% and are based on the assumption that one hospital recommendation will result in 15 prescriptions in primary care. An example of the cost effect of the policy is shown in chapter 6.

The NHS changes in 1989 included the concept of fundholding which gave budgets to GPs. If the drug component is exceeded then savings are expected from other parts of the budget. In reality, the health authority is required to meet any total overspend. For non-fundholders, each is set a budget for prescribing, which, if exceeded, results in reduced allocation at national level. The local effect is thus diluted and has little effect on local efforts to contain the costs.

In the latest White Paper, fundholding will be abolished and replaced with a system of locality purchasing in which one budget will be given and overspends will result directly in reduced funds for other purchasing.[5] Thus local hospitals will be directly affected by any overspends in primary care prescribing. This is likely to

mean that hospitals will have greater awareness of the cost of their recommended products in primary care and they are likely to be the prime movers in ensuring that their recommendations are evidence based and to consider the effect in primary care. It is also likely to result in reduced discounts from the pharmaceutical industry to hospitals.

The de-regulation of medicines

Self care, including the use of non-prescription medicines, is an important component of all health care systems.[67] In the UK in 1994 expenditure on such medicines by the public was £1.3 billion, equivalent to a third of the drugs bill. There are three legal categories of medicines in the UK: prescription only medicine (POM), pharmacy medicine (P), and general sales list (GSL). Prescription only medicines must be prescribed by a practitioner (mainly doctors and dentists). Pharmacy medicines must be sold by, or under the supervision of, a pharmacist and from a registered pharmacy outlet. General sales list medicines can be sold in both pharmacy and non-pharmacy premises and there is no requirement for professional supervision. Each country makes its own decisions about which medicines will be restricted to availability only on prescription.

The de-regulation of medicines to give wider availability should, it is argued, reduce health care costs in publicly funded systems. The theoretical basis is that the number of medical consultations will decrease, so fewer prescriptions will be written. There is little evidence, however, to demonstrate the impact of de-regulation or of the extent to which the use of de-regulated medicines substitutes for medical consultations, or simply delays them.[78] In the UK, there is evidence that those who pay for their prescriptions are more likely to purchase them.[9] The picture is not, however, straightforward and pricing policies, together with the likely period of use, are influencing factors. It is possible that de-regulation, with its associated advertising direct to the public, may increase the demand for certain medicines to be prescribed.

Concerns have been voiced about the potential safety problems arising from wider use of de-regulated medicines. This was particularly the case for H_2-receptor antagonists where it was thought that more serious conditions such as cancer might be masked. Studies in Denmark showed such fears to be unfounded.[10]

Nevertheless other medicines have been returned to prescription status where tighter controls on use have been deemed necessary in the interests of public safety.

Profit regulation

Since 1969, the UK Central Government directly conditions the profit that can be made on drugs sold to the NHS through the Pharmaceutical Price Regulation Scheme (PPRS).[11-13] This is a non-statutory scheme brokered between Central Government's Department of Health and the Association of the British Pharmaceutical Industry (ABPI), and its regulations apply to all drug companies whether or not they are members. The return on employed capital that drug companies can retain is 17–21% per annum. The objectives of the current scheme are:

- To secure the provision of safe and effective medicines at reasonable prices.
- To promote a strong and profitable pharmaceutical industry in the UK capable of such sustained research and development expenditure as should lead to the future availability of new and improved medicines.
- To encourage, in the UK, the efficient and competitive development and supply of medicines to pharmaceutical markets in this and other countries.

In 1994 the House of Commons Select Committee on Health recommended that the Department of Health supply Parliament with an annual report on the PPRS. In 1996, the first annual report was submitted to Parliament. In December 1997 the second report to Parliament showed that, in 1996, UK drug prices (ex-manufacturer prices) were on average higher than those in Italy or Spain, but lower than those in France, the Netherlands, and Germany. The analysis is based on 38 products available in each country. The report takes as a signal of success these reasonable prices. It is not, however, clear how representative the 38 products are of all products in each country, and analysis of prices paid, rather than manufacturers' prices, might yield a different picture.

There are serious problems with the scheme:

- No robust reason for the regulations.
- No theoretical basis.

- No empirical basis.
- A lack of transparency: it is not clear what happens in the scheme even though there is a European Union Directive, 89/105/EEC, against opaqueness in member states' policies affecting drug price and profit controls.
- A lack of accountability.
- A lack of due process: decision makers in Government do not explain their decisions to a wider audience.
- A shortage of impact analysis.
- No agreement on what is meant by "reasonable profits".
- Disincentives for international trade.
- Questions on its legality under European Union law.

It has been argued that prices can be reduced, if the political will exists to do so.[14] Not all are unique—some occur in other regulatory regimes such as reference pricing and "value for money" policies.

Management of prescribing by purchasers

Each health authority has a team, usually made up of both doctors and pharmacists, to develop a policy for medicines management. The lead role of prescribing policy and advice is usually given to the pharmacist(s) who have a daunting task. Their range of work encompasses policy making, identifying targets for change, the designing of incentive schemes, dealing with enquiries from GPs, as well as practice visits. The average health authority has one pharmacist. The other interested party in seeking prescribing change—the pharmaceutical industry—allocates rather more resources to its achievement. The industry is allowed to spend 9% of its total sales on advertising and most of this is directed to prescribers. On 1996 sales, this means the industry spent £409 million on advertising. As there are 124 health authorities, if each of them spent £100 000 per annum on prescribing advice then the industry spent 33 times more than the health authorities.

The Audit Commission reviewed prescribing practice in the UK and its main findings are the platform on which professional advisers and GPs seek to modify practice.[15]

The key areas in which savings could be made, with no loss of benefit to patients were identified as:

- Reducing overprescribing of certain drugs.
- Reducing the prescribing of drugs of limited clinical value.
- Substituting equally effective but less expensive drugs.
- Prescribing generic alternatives to proprietary brands.
- Using expensive preparations appropriately.

Incentive schemes for prescribing change are set in most health authorities and encouraged by the NHS Executive. It is very difficult to measure their effect, because there are many confounding factors, but one observational study suggested that incentive schemes achieved prescribing change in the required direction. This study suggested that non-fundholders respond to financial encouragement, as do fundholders.[16] The prescribing rate was identified by the Audit Commission as an area for more prudent prescribing and this target is set by some health authorities in incentive schemes—for example, to reduce the rate of prescribing antibiotics.

Generic prescribing is also a focus of interest in cost effective prescribing and the national average is now over 60%. One reason remains why prescribers hesitate to use generic products, although they recognise them to be a cost effective option. For non-computerised practices, the ability for prescribers to remember the long and complicated names of the generic equivalents are a real stumbling block to their use. Currently, active consideration is being given in the Department of Health to include, in a prescription form, *a tick the box* option in which a prescriber may write the brand name but tick to indicate that the generic option would be acceptable.

Fundholding has offered the opportunity to save costs on prescribing and to use those savings for practice development. As discussed in chapter 6, however, the results suggest that, as more practices become fundholding, differences in expenditure between them and non-fundholders are reduced.

Rising expectations

The fourth influence on the drugs bill is the rising expectations of health care professionals and patients. New drugs raise professional and personal expectations, and there is no national system to manage the introduction of new drugs. When a new drug comes on the market, it is massively promoted in the medical

press and increasingly in the mass media. What the NHS needs is a system to assess the clinical trial evidence, establish the numbers and types of patients who would benefit, estimate the merits of the drug in clinical and economic terms, and determine the resource implications. The West Midlands' way of introducing new drugs into primary care—the Midlands Therapeutic Review and Advisory Committee (MTRAC)—is described in chapter 9. A National Institute for Clinical Excellence (NICE) is to be set up. This body, independent of Government, will determine relative effectiveness and cost utility of drugs and novel clinical technologies.

International responses to rising drug costs

Concern about the rising allocation of resource to medicines is not a uniquely British phenomenon. All other health care systems, both government and insurance funded, have put in place measures to control the rate of increase. These are in two categories: controlling the cost and volume of prescribing, and seeking evidence of *value for money* by measurable outcomes and cost comparisons.

Europe

Extensive health care reforms have been introduced by European Union member states over the past two decades, largely in response to the need for cost containment. The main targets for reform have been on the supply side (purchasers, providers, and others involved in health care delivery such as pharmaceutical suppliers). The measures introduced have met with varying degrees of success and public acceptance. Action aimed at the demand side, for example increasing and extending cost sharing, has been less effective in controlling expenditure. Principal mechanisms used include:

- Introduction of overall budgets for health care expenditure (12 member states).
- Separation of purchasers and providers (the UK, Sweden, Spain—Catalonia and Basque regions—and Italy).
- Introduction of price competition between providers (Italy, the UK, Spain, the Netherlands, and Sweden).
- Capitation payment of first contact doctors (Ireland, Sweden, Germany [proposed]).

- Monitoring of what doctors authorise (Belgium and France). Germany and the Netherlands operate penalties for excessive prescribing.
- Introduction of a *limited list* (either positive or negative).
- Imposition of budget controls on pharmaceutical expenditure in addition to systems of influencing prices, for example, price control, profit control, or a reference price system (Belgium, Germany, Italy, the UK, France, and Spain).
- Development of a priority setting methodology and definition of services to be collectively funded (Spain, Sweden, Germany, the Netherlands, France).
- Several member states have shown interest in the appropriateness of health care interventions because a reduction in ineffective treatment may reduce health care costs without reducing health benefits.
- New forms of managed care include the development of practice and medical purchasing guidelines.

One of the main concerns of the European Union Commission in 1996 was to move towards the formation of a single European market for pharmaceuticals. Progress was, however, hampered by sovereignty of member states over pricing and reimbursement issues. Many governments introduced new pricing and reimbursement criteria, forcing drug prices down. The European Parliament adopted a resolution on an industrial policy for the pharmaceutical sector. This included proposals to allow generic companies to prepare for registration before patent/supplementary protection certificate expiry. The European Union Commission was asked to review the operation of the internal market with particular reference to the effects of the price transparency directive.

France

The Government began implementation of tough health care reforms, the main feature of which was a non-negotiable 2.1% ceiling on growth in drug expenditure in 1996. Strict prescribing guidelines were enforced. Other measures included reform of the hospital sector, restructuring of social security arrangements, and a requirement that there must be clear evidence of improved efficacy, reduced incidence of adverse effects, or a reduction in overall treatment costs before new products are reimbursed. A new Transparency Commission will be responsible for recommending

reimbursement status based on a medicoeconomic profile for each approved indication. The Government established a steering committee to monitor prescribing and consumption of medicines.

Germany

The Bundestag approved higher patient co-payments for drugs and a replacement of doctors' drug budgets by prescribing frameworks. New health purchasing models allow for competition among health care providers.

Italy

Parliament approved a *mini budget* including a reference pricing system and other measures to cut costs on drug expenditure. The Italian Drug Committee asked the Health Ministry for guidance on tackling the forecast deficit in the drug budget and warned of the impact of new products emerging from the European controlled registration system. Many were placed in *hospital only* or non-reimbursable categories. The potential role of private insurance is to be investigated.

Spain

To combat a substantial (12.5%) rise in drug expenditure, various policy changes were announced—promotion of generic prescribing, reference pricing, and a clamp down on prescription fraud. The pharmaceutical industry agreed to a payback agreement whereby a percentage of sales, where growth exceeded 2.6%, would be made.

Drug purchasers in Germany (since 1989), the Netherlands (since 1991), and Denmark (since 1993) have pricing control policies whereby the price they pay is related to a weighted basket of the products in the member states' market. Another alternative is to use an international basket of drugs as the reference base. Eire (since 1990) has used prices in Denmark, France, Germany, the Netherlands, and the UK as its reference base. Apart from France these countries have historically had the highest prices in the European Union. Portugal's reference price system used France, Spain, and Italy as the reference base, countries with historically lower drug prices. The authorities in Italy use a price setting system based on the average European price of the drug.

Such policies have attracted the attentions of market regulators at the European Union level. In May 1997 the European Union Commission argued that the Italian system may transgress the Treaty of Rome. In October 1997 the Italian authorities said that they would revisit their policies, but noted that the Italian drugs bill was exceeding the budget and that they had a duty to act as custodians of the Italian public purse.

The USA and Canada

Continued increase in health care costs continue to drive the expansion of managed care with more than 79% of American workers in such systems compared with 55% in 1992.

In Canada, the provincial governments have continued to introduce measures aimed at reducing prescription drug costs. Ontario became the last province to introduce patient co-payment for its benefit programme.

New Zealand

Pharmac, the drugs subsidy agency, was asked to make savings of $NZ28 million in the drugs budget, but stated that pharmaceutical expenditure would continue to grow at a *managed rate*. Concern was expressed that the forcing of lower prices for drugs would mean that New Zealand would no longer be a viable market for research based companies.

Value for money: a fourth hurdle?

A drug needs to have an official licence before it can be marketed. Three criteria are generally required: proof of the product's safety, efficacy, and quality. There is a growing interest in using a fourth hurdle: to prove the product is also good value for money.

In 1993 the Australian government ruled that, if a product wanted to be reimbursed on the Australian Pharmaceutical Benefits Scheme, proof that the drug was cost effective would be required. This policy was enacted even though drug prices in Australia were below the developed world average prices, and the Australian drugs bill was not rising faster than the world average. The Australian scheme remains the subject of intense debate.[17] There have been

calls in the UK for a similar scheme to be established and these are becoming louder as the drugs bill rises.

In November 1994 a set of national guidelines for the use of drugs economics was issued from the Canadian Co-ordinating Office for Health Technology Assessment. Since September 1995 applications to Ontario's provincial drugs reimbursement formulary have been considered incomplete if they do not include economic analysis of the drug in question. The national Canadian guidelines were intended to be the framework for provincial guidelines.

France and Norway are also showing considerable interest in mandating that drugs must be proven to be good value for money before they are considered for reimbursement. In late 1997, the Netherlands' new policy mandating that new drugs will only be considered for reimbursement once they have undergone cost effectiveness studies came to worldwide attention in medicines management, because the policy was put in place before the Dutch government had published guidelines for the cost effectiveness studies. To date few countries have emulated the Australian policy.

In 1997 the World Health Organization produced a draft working party document arguing that "sharper questions must be asked about (new products) final impact before any decision is taken on investing public funds in their use".[18] Essentially they are arguing for a fourth hurdle: prove the drug is good value for money or it will not be purchased.

Pharmaceutical company responses to rising expenditure

The pharmaceutical industry continues to be one of the most profitable sectors of the UK economy. It is likely to continue to be so, as the percentage of the elderly population rises, and as new and better drugs are developed. It knows, however, that decision making on the use of new drugs, particularly those of high unit cost, are now often made at health authority level and not by individual prescribers. This is likely to be reinforced by locality purchasers with one budget for all services. There will be increasing emphasis on *value for money* in decision making, which will require evidence of cost effectiveness, measurement of changes in the

quality of life, and closer scrutiny of how prices are arrived at. To achieve these outcomes, the industry will rightly expect greater clarity from purchasers on how these issues will be included in decision making.

The pharmaceutical industry already funds most clinical trials on medicines, and often, specific posts in centres in hospitals that use their products. The industry is also exploring its role in the concept of disease management, which originated in North America. Here the focus is the disease and its optimum cost effective management, rather than the drug acquisition costs alone. Such programmes have the potential to ensure higher and more consistent standards of care and that treatment and support are received in the most appropriate setting. They work by the implementation of clinical pathways of care, agreed by all the care givers, set standards for patient information, drug treatment protocols, and the timeliness of services, and define the caregivers and their training needs. Some health authorities are working on such care pathways, which will also be invaluable to locality purchasers. The pharmaceutical industry clearly has a potential role in some aspects of disease management. For example, their demonstrated ability in getting their message across to prescribers could be extended to the delivery of agreed patient education programmes on the disease and lifestyle changes as well as the optimum use of medicines.

Conclusion

This chapter has shown how expenditure on medicines will continue to rise and the underlying reasons.

There is a confusion of policies in the UK on medicines management—perhaps understandable because health systems have tried to respond to unprecedented rise in expenditure by reallocating budgets to primary care and to health authorities.

The UK pricing system, for now, looks unchallenging in containing costs compared with initiatives in other countries, and the time is ripe for a more rigorous examination of prices and measurement of the benefit of new drugs.

The pharmaceutical industry has every right to expect collaboration from health care systems in the development of policies for medicines use and, if criteria for clinical and cost effectiveness are shown, that new products will be used.

This chapter has tried to set the scene for the need for medicines management. The remaining chapters provide a review of the ways in which evidence can be assessed and then put into clinical practice.

1 Earl-Slater A, Bradley C. The inexorable rise in the National Health Service drugs bill: recent policies, future prospects. *Public Admin* 1996;**74**:393–411.
2 Office of Health Economics. *Compendium of health care statistics*, 10th edn. London: Office of Health Economics, 1997.
3 Office of National Statistics. *Population trends*. London: Office for National Statistics, 1997.
4 Marchant N. *Drivers of growth in medicines expenditure*. London: Office of Health Economics, 1997.
5 Department of Health. *The new NHS, modern, dependable*. London: HMSO, 1997.
6 Thomas DHV, Noyce P. The interface between the National Health Service and over the counter medicines. *BMJ* 1996;**312**:688–90.
7 Blenkinsopp A, Bradley C. Patients, society, and the increase in self-medication. *BMJ* 1996;**312**:629–32.
8 Ryan M, Yule B. Switching drugs from prescription only to over-the-counter availability: economic benefits in the United Kingdom. *Health Policy* 1990;**16**: 233–9.
9 Schaftheutle EI, Cantrill JA, Nicholson M, Noyce PR. Insights into the choice between self-medication and a doctor's prescription: a study of hayfever sufferers. *Int J Pharm Pract* 1996;**4**:156–61.
10 Anderson M, Schou JS. Are H_2 antagonists safe over the counter drugs? *BMJ* 1994;**309**:494.
11 Department of Health, Scottish Home and Health Department, Department of Health and Social Services Northern Ireland, the Welsh Office and the Association of the British Pharmaceutical Industry. *The agreement: pharmaceutical price regulation scheme*. London: HMSO, 1993.
12 International and Industry Division. *The pharmaceutical price regulation scheme: report to parliament*. London: Department of Health, 1996.
13 *Pharmaceutical prices regulation scheme. Second report to parliament*. London: Department of Health, 1997.
14 Earl-Slater A. Regulating the price of the United Kingdom's drugs: second thoughts after the government's first report. *BMJ* 1997;**314**:365–8.
15 Audit Commission. *A prescription for improvement—towards more rational prescribing health and personal services report*. London: HMSO, 1994.
16 Bateman DN, Campbell M, Donaldson LJ, Roberts SJ, Smith JM. A prescribing incentive scheme for non-fundholding general practices: an observational study. *BMJ* 1996;**313**:535–8.
17 Sloan FA, Grabowski HG. The impact of cost-effectiveness on public and private policies in health care: an international perspective. *Soc Sci Med* 1997; **45**:507–647.
18 World Health Organization. *Health for all for the 21st century—the health policy for Europe*. Denmark: WHO's Regional Committee, 1997.

5 Gathering and weighing the evidence

WENDY CLARK, JOHN MUCKLOW

Objectives

- To identify the place of evidence in the practice of medicine.
- To describe the rationale for evidence based medicine.
- To overview the strengths and weaknesses of an evidence based approach.
- To describe the practical process of evaluating the evidence in a structured manner.
- To discuss the limitations of evidence from clinical trials and meta-analyses.
- To clarify the role of the expert in the practice of evidence based medicine.

Evaluation of the clinical worth of health care interventions is an essential part of good medicine. During the last 30 years, however, continuous advances in clinical care have outpaced the incorporation of research evidence into clinical practice. Variations in the standard of practice among practitioners in both primary and secondary care have become more obvious with the growth of clinical audit. Questions are being asked about the reasons for this variation; the answers often lie in failure to adopt, or to adhere to, state of the art clinical procedures. It used to be said that it takes up to 10 years after first publication for a medical advance to become so established as to be commonplace. Now that public expectations of health care are so much higher, such cautious implementation of new developments is no longer acceptable. The clamour today is for clinical medicine to be increasingly *evidence based*. This chapter considers what this means, the assumptions

on which it is based, and the practicalities of gathering and weighing the evidence itself.

Evidence based medicine is a means of bringing the best evidence from clinical and health care research to bear when managing patients. It has been defined as "the conscientious and judicious use of current best evidence from clinical care research in the management of individual patients."[1] *Conscientious* because the evidence is applied consistently to each patient for whom it is relevant, and *judicious* because clinical expertise is necessary to balance the risks and benefits of diagnostic tests and alternative treatments for each patient, and to take into account his or her unique clinical circumstances, including baseline risk, co-morbid conditions, and preferences. *Current best evidence* means up to date guidance for which the research evidence is explicit.

The principles of evidence based medicine have been practised, though not widely, for over half a century. The concept has, however, recently been popularised and promoted in the belief that, by integrating medical education with clinical practice, and creating a clinical environment in which decisions are based on the best currently available evidence rather than on out of date training or anecdotal experiences with individual patients, it will improve the uniformity of patient care.

Although methodologically sound, the approach has critics as well as advocates. Some have argued that not all that is of value has been or can be measured in controlled clinical trials. Evidence based medicine takes considerable time both to learn and to practise, it provides information that is more applicable to populations than to individuals, and it takes little account of either the uncertainty inherent in clinical practice or economic issues. Its critics see evidence based medicine as a threat to clinical freedom because it holds medical literature to be more important than clinical experience.

The practice of evidence based medicine relies on systematic searching and evaluation of the published clinical and scientific literature. Detailed explanations on how to implement the techniques in everyday clinical practice can be found elsewhere.[2]

Gathering the evidence

The aim of searching the literature is to provide as comprehensive a list as possible of primary studies in the area under investigation.

Unfortunately, reliance on biomedical databases (for example, Medline, Excerpta Medica, Pharmline—see the end of the chapter) leads to incomplete retrieval of published studies because many articles are poorly indexed; such searches must be supplemented by skimming key journals in the relevant field and scanning the reference lists of retrieved articles. A new and increasingly useful literature source is the Cochrane Library, which contains both primary and secondary publications of clinical evidence, many of which have been independently and systematically evaluated.

Searchers need to be aware of bias in the reporting of clinical trials. A study describing a positive outcome for a new intervention is likely to feature widely in, for example, reports of sponsored meetings and sponsored journal supplements before it has been subjected to rigorous peer review. Reputable, independent, peer reviewed publications should be preferred as primary sources. The results of studies must be carefully compared to avoid considering multiple publications based on the same data.

Depending on the number of studies retrieved, it may be appropriate to restrict one's evaluation to those thought likely to give the most reliable results (Box 5.1). Amalgamations of published

---

Box 5.1　Hierarchy of evidence[3]

1　Strong evidence from at least one systematic review of multiple, well designed, randomised, controlled trials.

2　Strong evidence from at least one properly designed randomised controlled trial of appropriate size.

3　Evidence from well designed trials without randomisation, single group pre–post*, cohort, time series, or matched case control studies.

4　Evidence from well designed, non-experimental studies from more than one centre or research group.

5　Opinions of respected authorities, based on clinical experience, descriptive studies, and reports of expert committees.

*Evaluation of an intervention in a single group of patients where measurements are taken pre-intervention (baseline) and post intervention (end point) to identify the intervention effect.

---

studies can afford answers to a line of enquiry which are not apparent from single trials, and may reveal interpretations not apparent to the casual reader. There are two forms of amalgamation: systematic review and meta-analysis.

A systematic review is an overview of primary studies, which contains an explicit statement of objectives, materials, and methods, and has been conducted according to explicit and reproducible methodology. Such methodology limits bias and leads to more reliable and accurate conclusions than are usually generated by *expert* reviews—reviews compiled by one or more specialists in the field, drawing on selected published material to produce a particular interpretation. Systematic reviews enable a large amount of information to be assimilated quickly and indicate reasons for inconsistencies in results among different studies.

A meta-analysis (quantitative systematic review) is a mathematical synthesis of the results of two or more primary studies that address the same hypothesis in the same way. Although meta-analysis can increase the precision of a result it is important to ensure that the methods used for the review are valid and reliable. Reliance on an incomplete selection or the combination of results from heterogeneous trials will lead to erroneous conclusions. This has led to considerable criticism of this technique.

Weighing the evidence

The retrieved evidence must be examined carefully to assess its validity and clinical usefulness. This step is crucial, and is how one decides whether an article can be relied upon as a source of guidance. Unfortunately, publication alone is no guarantee of reliability, and too much published medical research is either lacking in methodological rigour or is irrelevant to the clinical questions one is likely to ask. Whether a study is published and where may be subject to the wishes of the sponsor or the author's affiliations, as well as the preferential publication of studies with positive outcomes (publication bias). The outcome of an intervention can be influenced by many factors other than the intervention itself. Confounding factors include the enthusiasm of the prescriber (prescriber bias), the expectations of the patient (patient bias), placebo effect, change in disease state with time, and within subject variability in clinical indices (regression to the mean). These factors can exaggerate the apparent response to an intervention such that observations made in poorly controlled trials tend to favour the intervention. Inadequate randomisation alone can lead to an overestimation of benefit by as much as 41%, whereas non-blind studies can overestimate benefit by up to 17%.[4]

The following are the aspects to consider when evaluating clinical trials.

Why was the study done, and what clinical questions were the authors addressing?

The introductory paragraph to a paper should state what the background to the research is, followed by a brief review of the literature. The hypothesis to be tested should be clearly stated.

How was the study done?

The study design should be appropriate to the research (Table 5.1). Although placebo controlled trials are required to prove efficacy, where trials compare two active drugs, the new drug should have been compared with the current standard therapy, at its standard dose. Unfortunately, it is not unusual to find new therapies compared with ineffective treatments or ineffective dosages. The methods section should identify what measures were taken to eliminate sources of bias and ensure the validity of the study results.

A reputable trial should be not only properly designed but also properly conducted. Poor trial discipline or protocol deviations—not always declared in the published version—will compromise the validity of the results.

Were the trial objectives appropriate?

Many clinical trials do not measure end points that are of direct clinical interest, but rely instead on indirect or surrogate end points. Where these are used they should be widely recognised as valid, reliable, and reproducible markers of response. For example, there is a large body of clinical trial evidence to suggest that the reduction of blood pressure prevents strokes and other direct complications of hypertension, but the correlation with ischaemic heart disease (IHD) events is less clear. As another example, the surrogate end point, changes in bone mineral density, is often measured when assessing treatment for osteoporosis, rather than the true end point of fracture rate. The true relationship between small changes in bone mineral density and fracture rates requires clarification.

Table 5.1 Application, advantages and disadvantages of different study designs

Type of study	Advantages and disadvantages	Uses
Case report Describes the medical history of a patient in the form of a story	*Advantages* Conveys a great deal of evidence that would be lost in a clinical trial or survey *Disadvantages* Quick and dirty—no control	Used to describe an unusual aspect of a disease, condition or an unanticipated adverse effect
Case–control study Observational study where the characteristics of subjects with a disease are compared with a selected group of control subjects without the disease	*Advantages* Sheds light on the cause of unexpected clinical events *Disadvantages* Validity depends on the appropriate selection of control subjects Cannot prove causality Cannot discover new events Cases need to be carefully allocated to avoid bias Bias is introduced by allocation and selection by outcome	Generally concerned with the aetiology of a disease rather than its treatment Often the only option for studying rare conditions
Cross sectional survey/study Interview or examination of a representative sample of subjects to gain answers to a clinical question at a given time	*Advantages* Can generate hypotheses about associations between risk factors and diseases *Disadvantages* Data are collected at a single time but may refer retrospectively to past experiences Cannot evaluate hypotheses	Used to identify opinions or quantify characteristics in a group of subjects

Cohort study Observational study of a group of subjects with a specific disease or characteristic who are followed up over a period of time	*Advantages* Can show causality as a result of the length of follow up Can estimate incidence *Disadvantages* Cannot discover rare events Can be prone to loss of subjects	Used to address questions relating to the events that occur in a group of patients over time
Randomised controlled trial (RCT) Patients are randomly allocated to a treatment by a validated process, followed up for a specified period and analysed in terms of outcomes defined at the outset	*Advantages* Allows rigorous evaluation of a single variable in a defined patient group Minimises bias *Disadvantages* Expensive and time consuming Can only address a small number of questions Not applicable to all interventions	Comparison of two or more interventions under controlled conditions in a predefined patient group
Parallel group Patients are randomised to active or control treatment	*Advantages* The most rigorous form of RCT *Disadvantages* Groups must be comparable at baseline Only a proportion of patients receive active treatment	Appropriate for curative treatments
Crossover study Controlled trial where each patient acts as their own control	*Advantages* Each patient acts as their own control *Disadvantages* The variable measured must be stable over time and adequate washout periods given between two treatments to avoid biases and carry over effects Long studies will be required for slow acting treatments	Only appropriate for evaluating palliative treatments of chronic stable conditions Useful for rare conditions Not suitable for acute treatments

The measurement of symptomatic effects, functional effects, psychological effects, or social effects is difficult. The outcome measure used in these areas should have been objectively validated, to confirm that the scale used measures what it is purported to measure and that changes in this outcome measure adequately reflect changes in the status of the patient. For symptomatic scales it is important to know who reported the effect, patient or clinician, because this could change the emphasis of the reported results. The method by which these data are elicited can also affect the results—open reporting is subject to the least bias.

The data collected for these end points can be subjective or objective. Objective data are to be preferred because they are less prone to bias.

What were the results?

It is important that all the patients entered into the trial are accounted for at the end, with the outcome of withdrawn patients discussed. A basic schematic trial profile is shown in Fig 5.1; this can be used to map the trial.

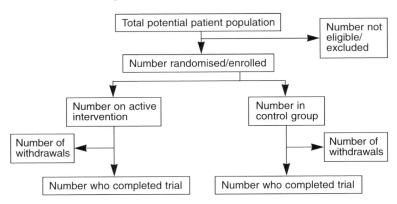

Figure 5.1   Basic trial profile

The results described should answer the questions posed at the outset. Occasionally a secondary end point becomes the main focus of the analysis and discussion because it has shown a favourable effect of the study intervention. The results of such an analysis should be viewed with caution: they may be less valid than those relating to the primary end point which the study was specifically

designed to explore. Similar criticisms can also be applied to subgroup analyses that were not originally planned. If a set of data is analysed and reanalysed often enough a positive result can arise purely by chance. Such *data dredging* may point to the need for further investigation in a subset of patients, but cannot be relied upon as a source of evidence.

How were the results presented?

Randomised trials provide not only qualitative conclusions about whether an intervention is better but also quantitative estimates of the extent to which it is better. But the way the results are presented can mislead. Study results often present the relative benefit of an active treatment over the reference comparator as the relative risk, the relative risk reduction, or the odds ratio. These measures are used extensively in both clinical and epidemiological investigations, but give no indication of the underlying incidence of the event being prevented. For example, a relative risk reduction of 50% could relate to 50 out of a projected 100 events per 1000 patients treated being prevented or only five out of a projected 10. By contrast, absolute risk reductions consider the reduction in risk in the context of the underlying incidence of the event being prevented. For clinical decision making, the reciprocal of the absolute risk reduction, the *number needed to treat* (NNT), is even more meaningful. The measure identifies the number of patients who need to be treated in order for one person to obtain the required outcome. It conveys both statistical and clinical significance to the doctor. Furthermore, it can be used to extrapolate published findings to a patient with an arbitrary specified baseline risk when the relative risk reduction associated with treatment is constant for all levels of risk. The principles can be used to calculate number of lives saved (Table 5.2).

Was the statistical analysis appropriate?

The statistical tests used to analyse the trial findings should be scrutinised to assess their appropriateness and hence the validity of the conclusions. Statistical analyses are considered to be more robust if they are conducted on an intention to treat basis, where data are included from all patients, even those who did not complete

Table 5.2 Equivalent figures for absolute risk reduction and numbers needed to treat for the examples given in the text

Group	Number	Events	Relative risk reduction (%)	Absolute risk reduction (%)	NNT
Treatment	1000	50	50	5	20
Control	1000	100			
Treatment	1000	5	50	0.5	200
Control	1000	10			

the study. This more closely approaches the real life situation where some patients are not compliant with therapy.

No statistical test can definitely *prove* anything. These tests serve merely to quantify the likelihood that the observed result is a real effect and has not arisen by chance. Although p values are useful, they should be considered along with the confidence intervals around the result. A large confidence interval, including zero, suggests that the trial is too small and uninformative, whereas a very narrow confidence interval completely shifted away from zero suggests that the treatment effect is both statistically and clinically significant.

How was safety assessed?

When assessing the safety of an intervention, the number of patients in whom the intervention has been trialled and the range of adverse events seen are of paramount importance. The 95% confidence limits for the true frequency of a particular adverse event in a clinical trial in which no such event occurs lie between zero and $3/n$, where n is the sample size. Thus, if no cases are observed in a study of 300 patients, one can be 95% confident only that the true frequency does not exceed 1% ($3/300$). A further confounder is the events background incidence of the adverse event. A high background incidence of competing adverse events greatly increases the number of patients who need to be treated with the intervention before an association with the drug can be inferred. Rare adverse events that have a low background incidence also require exposure to relatively large patient numbers for detection.

The method used to collect reports of adverse events can influence the results obtained. Closed questions or suggestions, or

prior beliefs, may lead the trial participants/investigators to look for or report only selective adverse events.

What did the authors conclude?

The discussion section of a paper should be a methodological review of the results that leads logically to the authors' conclusions. It should account for any observed inconsistencies in, or shortcomings of, the study in a satisfactory way.

Once all these points have been considered, a final conclusion about the usefulness of the study must be made. The results of statistical tests must be taken into account along with a clinical judgment as to whether they represent a clinically useful outcome. A checklist to aid in the evaluation of these criteria is given in Box 5.2.

Limitations of the evidence

Clinical trials give us an indication of the outcomes that can be expected when an intervention is used in a defined way in a specified group of recipients. This artificial environment cannot, however, provide us with all the information we need before using the intervention. Patients recruited to trials of new drugs are often unrepresentative because of extensive exclusions and entry restrictions on grounds of age, weight, renal function, child bearing potential, previous treatment experience, concomitant treatment, alcohol use, compliance, and so on. This overprotective attitude to new drugs may result in unexpected problems after licensing, such as unforeseen toxicity in elderly people. A notable, if not extreme, example of this was flosequinan, launched in 1992 in the UK for the treatment of heart failure in elderly people; a study published after the launch of the product identified that this treatment was associated with increased mortality and the product was subsequently withdrawn.

The evidence from scientific assessments of treatments for rare diseases can also be very limited. The number of patients with the disease is often too small to allow the treatment to be evaluated with scientific rigour. Patient baseline characteristics are likely to be more diverse than when studying a treatment for a common condition. Treatments for rare diseases often have to be studied in multinational trials, which lead to such variation in both the

Box 5.2   Critical appraisal checklist to evaluate a therapy article

	Yes	No	Unclear
Is the journal reputable—refereed?	☐	☐	☐
Was it an independent investigation?	☐	☐	☐
Are the authors well recognised experts in the field?	☐	☐	☐
Why was the study done?			
Was the aim of the study explicit?	☐	☐	☐
How was the study done?			
Was the trial design appropriate?	☐	☐	☐
Was the trial duration suitable?	☐	☐	☐
Were sufficient numbers of patients studied to make the results credible?	☐	☐	☐
Were the exclusion and inclusion criteria explicit and appropriate?	☐	☐	☐
Were the control and treatment groups comparable at entry?	☐	☐	☐
Were patients, health workers, and study personnel blinded to treatment?	☐	☐	☐
Was the assignment of patients to treatment randomised?	☐	☐	☐

	Yes	No	Unclear
Aside from the intervention, were the groups treated equally?	☐	☐	☐
For comparative trials			
1. Were appropriate comparative treatments chosen	☐ ☐	☐ ☐	☐ ☐
2. Were appropriate doses used?			
Was patient compliance with the intervention measured or controlled?	☐	☐	☐
Is there evidence of good trial discipline?			
Were the trial end points appropriate?			
Were these clearly defined?	☐ ☐	☐ ☐	☐ ☐
Were these well recognised markers of response?			
Were all clinically important outcomes considered?	☐	☐	☐
Was the measurement of end-points appropriately standardised?	☐	☐	☐
What were the results?			
Were all patients who entered the trial accounted for at the end?	☐	☐	☐
Were the outcomes of people who withdrew described?	☐	☐	☐

Box 5.2 *continued*

Yes ☐ No ☐ Unclear ☐

- Were the results numerically consistent? ☐ ☐ ☐
- Was follow-up complete? ☐ ☐ ☐
- Were patients analysed in the group to which they were randomised? ☐ ☐ ☐
- Did the results answer the study question? ☐ ☐ ☐
- Was post-hoc subgroup analysis conducted? ☐ ☐ ☐

How were the results presented?
- Was the treatment effect large in real terms? ☐ ☐ ☐
- Was this clinically significant? ☐ ☐ ☐
- Was the treatment effect precise? ☐ ☐ ☐
- Can the NNT be calculated from the data presented? ☐ ☐ ☐

Was the statistical analysis appropriate?
- Was a statistician cited as an author? ☐ ☐ ☐
- Did the authors use appropriate statistical tests? ☐ ☐ ☐
- If the authors used obscure statistical tests:
  1. Have they stated why? ☐ ☐ ☐
  2. Have they referenced them? ☐ ☐ ☐

Yes ☐ No ☐ Unclear ☐

Was the statistical analysis done on an intention to treat basis?
- Were p values calculated and interpreted correctly? ☐ ☐ ☐
- Were confidence intervals calculated? ☐ ☐ ☐
- Did the confidence intervals include zero? ☐ ☐ ☐
- Did the confidence intervals overlap between the two treatments? ☐ ☐ ☐
- Were significant effects confined to post-hoc subgroup analysis? ☐ ☐ ☐

How was safety assessed?
- Were adverse events recorded "openly" by patients? ☐ ☐ ☐
- Are adverse events described and related to drop outs? ☐ ☐ ☐

What did the authors conclude?
- Were the authors' conclusions justified by their data? ☐ ☐ ☐
- Did the discussion account for any observed inconsistencies? ☐ ☐ ☐
- Were the effects of the intervention expressed in terms of the likely benefit or harm, which an individual patient could expect? ☐ ☐ ☐

conduct of study and the interpretation/evaluation of end points by study investigators, that they preclude pooled analysis. The understandable demand, among patients with conditions for which there was previously no therapeutic option, for treatments to be made rapidly and widely available puts great pressure on drug regulators, and can be difficult to resist. Such accelerated use, before the completion of good quality studies, reduces the evidence base supporting the product and increases the likelihood of unforeseen problems.

The place of expert judgment—putting it all together

An examination of the published literature about a particular intervention, however thorough, may not allow one to state with confidence what its place should be in everyday clinical practice. This requires a value judgment by an expert in the relevant specialist field, proficient in the treatment of patients with the condition in question, who understands the benefits and limitations of existing therapy well enough to put in context the relative efficacy and safety of the new product. The expert can advise on which patients are likely to benefit most, the gains they can expect, the anticipated adverse events, and any monitoring required. Few new chemical entities are so much more effective, or so much safer, than existing products that they can be recommended for widespread use immediately. Such hubris often leads to regret, either because initial promise is not fulfilled or because widespread use reveals a serious adverse event not previously apparent. The expertise of the specialist charged with advising on the place of a new drug lies in targeting the drug's use at an early stage, so that it reaches patients in whom the benefit–risk ratio is greatest and is withheld from those for whom it offers only a slight advantage over existing treatments.

Conclusions

- Evidence based medicine is a valuable tool that allows the most recent findings of clinical and health care research to influence individual patient care.
- The evidence is gathered from a comprehensive search of the literature, facilitated increasingly by developments in information technology, and by professional analyses of published research.

- The evidence must then be weighed by assessing why and how each study was done, how the results were presented and analysed, and how the authors interpreted their findings. Greatest reliance should be placed on randomised controlled trials, analysed on an intention to treat basis, which result in a quantitative estimate of individual patient benefit and/or risk.
- Systematic reviews and meta-analyses may save the searcher much time and effort but should not be viewed uncritically.
- The results of clinical trials cannot be extrapolated directly to everyday clinical practice because the patients studied may be unrepresentative and the setting artificial. Studies of treatments for rare diseases present particular problems.
- Introducing the evidence into clinical practice requires expert judgment, especially when interpreting its significance for others.

Further reading

Anon. An introduction to assessing medical literature. *MEREC Briefing* 1995;**9**: 1–8.

Greenhalgh T. *How to read a paper: the basics of evidence-based medicine.* London: BMJ Publishing Group, 1997.

McInnes G, Murray G. Design and analysis of clinical trials. *Prescribers J* 1991;**31**: 227–34.

NHS Centre for Reviews and Dissemination. *Undertaking systematic reviews of research effectiveness.* CRD Report 4. York: University of York, 1996.

Ramsay L, Yeo W. Critical appraisal of clinical trials. *Prescribers J* 1991;**31**:250–7.

Rosenberg W, Donald A. Evidence-based medicine: an approach to clinical problem solving. *BMJ* 1995;**310**:1122–6.

Biomedical databases on the internet

Medline: http://www.ncbi.nlm.nih.gov/PubMed

Excerpta Medica: http://www.healthgate.com/HealthGate/price/embase.html

Cochrane database of systematic reviews: http://www.cochrane.co.uk

The Cochrane Library is available on CD ROM or disk from the BMJ Publishing Group, PO Box 295, London WC1H 9TE. Tel: 0171 383 6185/6245; fax: 0171 383 6662.

1 Sackett DL, Rosenberg W, Gray JA, Haynes RB, Richardson WS. Evidence-based medicine: what it is and what it isn't. *BMJ* 1996;**312**:71–2.
2 Sackett DL, Richardson WS, Rosenberg W, Haynes RB. *Evidence-based medicine: how to practice and teach EBM*. London: Churchill Livingstone, 1997.
3 Moore A, McQuay H. Type and strength of efficacy evidence. *Bandolier* 1997; 4:8.
4 Moore A. Drug information and evidence-based medicine. *UK Drug Information Conference Proceedings* 1996;**3**:112–14.

6 Issues and directions in prescribing analysis

MARTIN FRISCHER, STEPHEN CHAPMAN

Objectives

- Define the nature and scope of prescribing analysis.
- Describe the strengths and limitations of available data, for example, prescription items and defined daily doses.
- Show how Prescribing Analysis and Cost (PACT) data can be used to interpret the market, to monitor change, and to identify unusual patterns of prescribing.
- Identify future data developments, for example, electronic data interchange and expert prescribing systems.
- Review studies of prescribing variation in relation to factors such as morbidity, age, deprivation, general practitioner fundholding.
- Consider how doctors' and patients' beliefs and attitudes towards medicines relate to prescribing.
- Outline new methods for analysing prescribing data, for example, bayesian inference, multilevel modelling, and geographical information systems.

Issues in prescribing analysis

With increasing levels of prescribing in the UK,[1] there is growing pressure to make effective use of prescribing data in order to inform policy[2] and to ensure equitable distribution of resources.[3] The inherent complexity of prescribing data means, however, that most large scale analysis has hitherto focused on readily available measures such as the number of items prescribed or

the total cost. Although analyses based on such measures are useful for certain purposes, they do not consider prescribing in terms of volume, patients, or morbidity, and are therefore susceptible to misinterpretation. Thus, comparing regions within the UK in terms of number of prescriptions is hazardous because the quantity of drugs prescribed is not known. If total cost of drugs prescribed is used to assess regional variation, difficulties arise because of variation in morbidity, demographic characteristics, and changes in drug prices. Many analyses focus on particular drugs and are primarily economic in nature. For example, if prescribing for a particular drug is changed from proprietary to generic then a given amount will be saved. Although qualitative research has highlighted the complexity of prescribing decisions made by patients and doctors,[5] insights from this area of research are rarely combined with quantitative aspects of prescribing.

Whether prescribing could be improved depends on the standards by which current prescribing is judged. In 1973, Parish stated that good prescribing should "be appropriate, safe, effective and economic".[4] Views of prescribing have, however, changed and there is now more emphasis on concordance between prescriber and patient rather than patient compliance to the prescriber's decision.[6] Barber[7] proposed that good prescribing should aim to "maximise effectiveness, minimise risks, minimise costs and respect patient choices". Thus, although the increase in generic prescribing in recent years might be in accordance with the 1973 definition, it may conflict with the more recent view if, for example, patients were unhappy about switching from a proprietary to a generic formulation.

Interpretation of prescribing data is complicated because there are many indicators that can be derived from routinely collected data. Indicators may be based on pharmacological properties, cost, and practice characteristics and from these a range of ratios can be derived. Harris[8] observed, however, that there are few areas in which standards can be confidently set. One reason is that, although prescribing is assumed to reflect morbidity, standard indicators are based solely on dispensed prescriptions without reference to underlying medical conditions. The potential to change this situation has recently changed with databases that have high quality prescribing and diagnostic information.[9]

Prescribing data

Prescribing Analysis and Cost data

The basic unit of prescribing analysis is the prescription and, for practical purposes, data on dispensed prescriptions in primary care are the usual starting point for analysis. Each prescription contains information on substance, dosage, and quantity. Prescription data are aggregated by the Prescription Pricing Authority (PPA) and national summary tables are published by the Department of Health in the *Statistical Bulletin* series.[1] The PPA produces more detailed information for general practitioners and other health professionals in the PACT report. Some of the main features of the PACT report at practice level are shown in Box 6.1.

Box 6.1   Main features of Prescribing Analysis and Cost (PACT) report at practice level

Comparison of practice's total prescribing costs with health authorities (HAs) and national equivalent practices. The comparative practices are weighted so as to be of the same size and with the same proportion of patients aged 65 and over.

Practice costs broken down into therapeutic areas. The 20 leading cost drugs in the practice are summarised in terms of the number of prescriptions, total cost, proportion of practice's total cost, and change from last year. Proprietary names with generic equivalents are highlighted.

Number of items prescribed by the practice compared with the HA and national equivalents and the proportion of items written and dispensed generically.

There are a range of other analyses, for example: (1) average cost per item within therapeutic areas and comparison with health authority and national equivalents; (2) changes in practice prescribing costs over last eight quarters; (3) individual practices' own top 40 sections of the *British National Formulary* in terms of cost.

These analyses enable practices to monitor their prescribing and assess various issues, for example: compare proportion of items prescribed generically to health authority and national averages; identify therapeutic sections that account for largest proportion of

spending; consider whether prescribing in the most expensive areas is rational.[10]

At national level, PACT data provide information on overall trends and breakdown by therapeutic categories, drug groups, and regions.[1] Between 1995 and 1996 the net ingredient cost (NIC) of prescription items rose by £326 million to £4007 million in England alone, an increase of 8.9%, and the number of prescription items increased to 485 million, an increase of 2.4%. Central nervous system disorders rose from fourth to third in the ranking of therapeutic groups. The largest increase in prescription items was for cardiovascular disease which increased by 6 million to 91 million in 1996. For drug groups, the largest increase in cost was for antidepressant drugs, which increased by £33 million to £191 million. This group also had the largest increase in the volume of prescriptions, up 2 million to 15 million, an increase of 13%. There is considerable variation in drug spending within England. The average NIC per head in England was £81.68, ranging from £100.22 in Sunderland to £68.55 in north and mid-Hampshire. The average NIC per prescription was £8.26 in England, ranging from £10.23 in Kensington, Westminster, and Chelsea, to £6.87 in Sheffield.

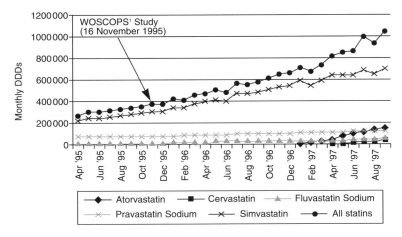

Figure 6.1 Defined daily doses of statins
1. WOSCOPS—West of Scotland Coronary Prevention Study Group. West of Scotland Coronary Prevention Study: Identification of high-risk groups and comparison with other cardiovascular intervention trials. Lancet 1996;**384**:1339–42.
Source: Keele University prescribing analysis. Prescription Pricing Authority data

PACT analyses can be used to interpret the market, monitor key changes and alert health authorities and their prescribing advisers to any unusual patterns of prescribing.

Figure 6.1 shows how published research can change prescribing. Initial uptake of statin prescribing for reducing cholesterol was relatively low, but increased following publications of two major clinical trials in 1994 and 1995.[11][12]

PACT data also help to monitor the impact of warnings about drugs. Figure 6.2 shows how prescribing of third generation oral

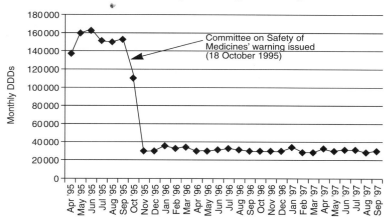

Figure 6.2 Prescribing of third generation contraceptives following the Committee on Safety of Medicines' warning
Source: Keele University prescribing analysis. Prescription Pricing Authority data

contraceptives dropped after the Committee on Safety of Medicines issued a warning. Figure 6.3 shows the effect of a paper published in the *British Medical Journal* warning of the potential side effects of minocycline.

Cost comparisons show the relatively high unit cost of sophisticated delivery systems. In Fig 6.4 we see a relatively low rate of prescribing for Diskhalers for asthma, the more sophisticated system, and similarly for the hormone replacement therapy patches in Fig 6.5.

PACT data are useful as a management tool when considering performance management of health authorities. Figure 6.6 shows the disproportionate use of buccal formulations of glyceryl trinitrate tablets in one health authority. Further investigation highlighted the role of one hospital which used buccal formulations, but did

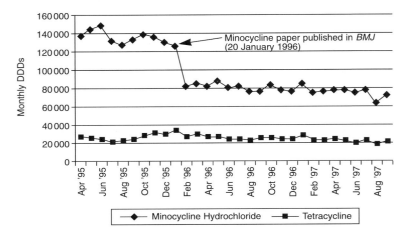

Figure 6.3 Prescribing of minocycline and tetracycline following publication of warning in the British Medical Journal.
Source: Keele University prescribing analysis. Prescription Pricing Authority data.

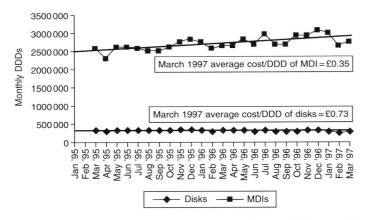

Figure 6.4 Prescribing of beclomethasone metered dose inhalers (MDIs) and disks in relation to cost
Source: Keele University prescribing analysis. Prescription Pricing Authority data.

not ensure that discharged patients received standard preparations when returning to primary care.

Figure 6.7 shows the high usage of finasteride in one health authority. Further investigation revealed that prescribing rose after a drug company sponsored trial in a local hospital.

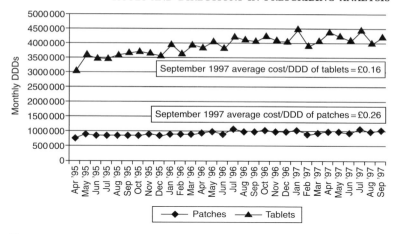

Figure 6.5   Prescribing of hormone replacement therapy delivery systems in relation to cost
Source: Keele University prescribing analysis. Prescription Pricing Authority data.

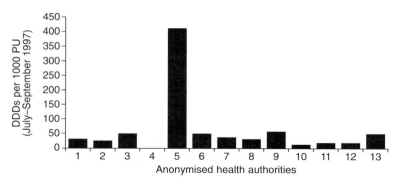

Figure 6.6   Variation in glyceryl trinitrate (buccal tablets only), defined daily doses per 1000 prescribing units, July to September 1997
Source: Keele University prescribing analysis. Prescription Pricing Authority data.

Prescribing units

Any comparative analysis of PACT data needs to be treated with caution because the units of comparison may not be the same. Regions vary by age/sex structure, deprivation, ethnicity, and morbidity, while practices will have further variation in terms of resources and GP characteristics. To facilitate more meaningful comparisons, an adjustment was made to PACT data via the prescribing unit (PU) where patients aged 65 and over count as 3

81

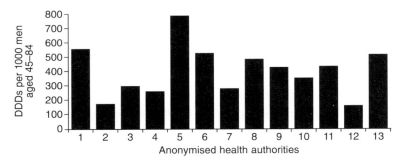

Figure 6.7   Variation in finasteride defined daily doses per 1000 prescribing units, July to September 1997
Source: Keele University prescribing analysis. Prescription Pricing Authority data.

PUs. This adjustment was justified on the assumption that patients in this age group require, on average, three times as many prescriptions as those aged under 65. It has long been recognised that the PU is not very sensitive[13] and in 1993 a new weighting factor was developed.[14] The ASTRO-PU (age, sex and temporary resident originated prescribing unit) weights for nine age bands for males and females, and for temporary residents, and this is now used in the setting of prescribing budgets.[15] More recently weightings for specific therapeutic groups have been established because the use of therapeutic drug groups varies by age and sex distributions, for example. Cardiovascular and gastrointestinal drug prescribing is more prevalent among older patients, whereas antibiotic prescribing is similar for all age/sex groups. These weightings are called STAR-PUs (specific therapeutic group age/sex related prescribing units) and have been developed for eight therapeutic groups, which account for 85% of prescribing in England.[15]

Prescription items and defined daily doses

Although many prescribing analyses are concerned with volume, the validity of the prescribing item has been called into question. Bogle and Harris[16] point out that the number of items is unsatisfactory as an index of volume because it does not specify the quantity of prescribed medication, for example, number of

tablets or millilitres of liquid. They examined variation in the average quantity per item of ten commonly prescribed drugs across practices, Family Health Service Authorities, and regions. All drugs had wide variation, for example, for atenolol 100 mg tablets, the number ranged from five to 366. Two quantities, 28 and 56 tablets, corresponding to four and eight weeks' supply, accounted for 77% of prescribed items. Thus, even when only two quantities are prescribed, one practice might be prescribing twice as much as another for a given number of items. As variability was not found to diminish at Family Health Service Authority or regional level, it would appear that the item is a poor measure of volume, and that it would be better to use a measure that takes account of the actual volume of drug prescribed.

A more accurate index of prescribing volume is the defined daily dose (DDD). A DDD is the typical adult maintenance dose of a drug per day as defined by the World Health Organization.[17] Thus, if information on the quantity of drug prescribed is available, the number of DDDs can be calculated. There are, however, several problems with DDDs.[8] First, not all drugs have them, for example, skin preparations and paediatric doses. Second, DDDs are international units and different countries may use the same drug in different ways. Third, some DDDs are set at the dosages used in hospital and may be higher than those prescribed by GPs. Finally, DDDs are only updated once every 10 years. In England, an expert group was convened to produce average daily quantities (ADQs) which more accurately reflect British GPs' prescribing.[18]

Although the DDD is superior to the item as a unit of comparative analysis, difficulties may arise when they are used in estimating disease prevalence because DDDs correspond to a drug's principal indication. As most drugs have multiple indications, using DDDs will inflate prevalence estimates as the drug will be prescribed for other conditions. In a study of three drugs used in treating heart disease, Clarke et al[19] found that there was considerable variation in average prescribed daily doses in five practices in Nottingham (Table 6.1). DDDs were found to correspond to the median dose of frusemide. Use of the median dose in the estimation of the prevalence of heart failure and angina results produced a rate of 5.2 out of 1000, although use of the mean dose resulted in a rate of 7.8 out of 1000, a difference of 50%. In a refined version of this analysis, however, Clarke et al[20] advise that PACT data can

Table 6.1   Comparison of DDDs and actual usage of three drugs used in treatment of heart disease

Drug	DDD	Actual range	Mean	Median
Sublingual glyceryl trinitrate (tablets)	5	1–34	2.3	1.5
Frusemide (mg)	40	20–1000	60	40
Isosorbide (mg)	60	20–120	47.6	40

Source: Clarke *et al*, 1994.[19]

be used to determine disease prevalence for drugs with specific indications.

Prescribing and morbidity in general practice

One way of circumventing the limitations of PACT data is to use a database containing both prescribing and diagnostic data. The UK General Practice Research Database (GPRD) contains such information and currently receives data from 525 practices with a population of 3.4 million patients and over 30 million years of prescribing histories.[21] All participating GPs are required to record every prescription and all significant morbidity. The Office for National Statistics[22] publishes morbidity and prescription rates by *British National Formulary* chapter, age, sex, and region. The database can also be analysed to provide information on patients with selected diseases prescribed specific drugs (Table 6.2).

Table 6.2   Epidemiological data on patients with treated asthma

	Male	Female
Patient numbers	1 408 338	1 464 876
Number of asthma patients	90 704	93 530
Prevalence rate per 1000 registered patients	64.4	63.8
Percentage prescribed corticosteroids	62.4	66.6

Source: West Midlands General Practice Research Database, 1994.

Although the GPRD indicates that there is regional variation in treated asthma across England (for example, in 71.2 out of 1000 patients in Mersey compared with 44.7 out of 1000 in south-east Thames), the database itself can only be used to explore a limited set of patient and GP characteristics. There are, for example, no data on patients' socioeconomic status. It can be used, however,

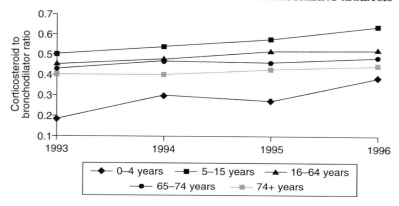

Figure 6.8   Ratio of corticosteroid to bronchodilator medication in the West Midlands, 1993–1996
Source: Keele University prescribing analysis. General Practice Research Database data.

to explore other aspects of asthma therapy such as the ratio of prophylaxis (corticosteroid) to bronchodilator medication. The general increase in the ratio (Fig 6.8) may be attributable to new guidelines on the management of asthma which were introduced in 1993.[23]

Although GPRD diagnoses are based solely on clinical judgment, several studies have found them to be reliable and accurate when compared to a number of other sources, for example, consultants' letters, hospital discharge letters, and questionnaire responses from GPs.[24][25] Nazareth et al[26] found that the sensitivity, specificity, and predictive value of diagnoses for schizophrenia and non-affective psychosis were good in a sample of 13 London practices. Furthermore, prescribing information was found to be more complete on computer than on paper records.

Figure 6.9 shows the results of an exploratory analysis which sought to investigate the extent to which prescribing for duodenal disease was influenced by date of diagnosis or the currently recommended treatment. In 1991 and 1992 all patients were treated with H_2-receptor antagonists which at that time was the most appropriate treatment. By 1995, however, most patients had been switched to the now recommended proton pump inhibitors. These findings suggest that, at least for duodenal disease, date of diagnosis does not appear to have much impact on current prescribing.

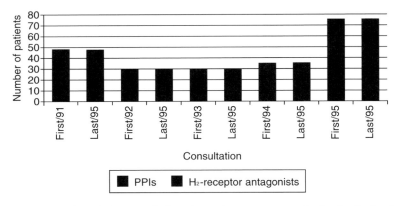

Figure 6.9 Type of drug prescribed at first and most recent consultation for duodenal disease
Source: Keele University prescribing analysis. General Practice Research Database data.

The other main source of information on morbidity in general practice is the National Morbidity Survey which is conducted every 10 years in England and Wales.[27] The fourth survey was conducted from September 1991 to August 1992. Sixty practices with 500 000 registered patients recorded diagnoses for every face to face GP–patient contact. Detailed sociodemographic information was also recorded for patients. Of registered patients 78% consulted their GP compared with 71% in 1981–82. Trends in patient consulting rate for asthma are shown in Fig 6.10.

The National Morbidity Survey does not contain information on prescribing, but the morbidity by sex, age group, and socioeconomic characteristics from the sample can be applied to the demographic structure of any population to provide estimates of expected morbidity. It could potentially be used in many areas of prescribing research, which currently use surrogates of morbidity such as deprivation indices. Hollowell[21] reports good concordance between the GPRD and the National Morbidity Survey for selected diagnoses.

Future electronic developments

The advent of electronic PACT data has already had a considerable impact on prescribing analysis. Within the next 5–10 years there will be further developments centring on electronic

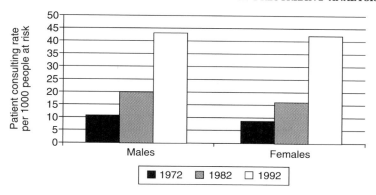

Figure 6.10 Patient consulting rate for asthma (per 1000 people at risk), England and Wales
Source: National Morbidity Survey data.[27]

data interchange (EDI) which, unlike PACT, will be patient based and comprise complete medication profiles with information on prescription quantities, frequencies, and durations. Various scenarios are being considered, involving transmission of electronic prescription records directly from GPs to pharmacies or indirectly via the PPA; the PPA would also receive electronic dispensing records from pharmacies.[28] These electronic records will contain a patient identifier code that will enable, for example, comparison of drugs prescribed and drugs dispensed. A further step might involve using EDI to evaluate expert systems such as PRODIGY (prescribing rationally with decision support in general practice study), which are currently being developed to provide on screen advice to GPs on treatment options.[29]

Prescribing analysis

Prescribing at practice level

Given the concerns about the emphasis placed on cost indicators in prescribing analysis, there has been considerable research into developing more sophisticated measures using PACT data. Bateman *et al*[30] suggest 13 new measures, developed after qualitative and quantitative research with GPs. A consensus group identified four areas: (1) overall generic prescribing rate; (2) choice

of drug within a therapeutic group; (3) drugs with limited clinical value; and (4) therapeutic areas where the volume of prescribing might indicate good or bad prescribing. The group rejected several commonly suggested markers of quality, for example, ratio of inhaled steroids to bronchodilators in asthma treatment, because there is no agreement about how much prescribing meets the needs of asthmatic patients and because prescribing patterns are changing rapidly. From the 13 measures, scores from − 1 (*good*) to 14 (*bad*) were derived for the 518 practices in the Northern Regional Health Authority. Fundholding practices were generally low scoring but there were no differences in terms of dispensing status. Although this methodology has wide applicability, there are a number of issues that require further research, for example, how many measures are needed for each therapeutic area? It also remains to be seen whether the scoring system requires adaptation to take account of local population needs. Other small scale studies have identified specific prescribing measures, for example, Catford[31] found that 42% of a sample of 72 GPs in Wessex had prescribed a hazardous or undesirable drug for children in a single month.

A frequent aim in prescribing analysis is to explain variation in prescription rates and costs. In a study of all the 98 Family Health Service Authorities in England and Wales in 1987, Forster and Frost[32] looked at the total number of prescriptions and total costs from a 1/200 sample of prescriptions in relation to practices' age/sex structure, overall standardised mortality ratio (SMR), Jarman score, and the number of general practice principals per 100 population. Using multiple regression techniques they found that age and sex explained 51% of the variation in prescription rates, whereas adding SMR, Jarman, and GP principals increased the variance explained to 65%. For prescription costs per patient, age/sex structure explained 44% of the variance; adding SMR, Jarman, and number of GP principals increased the proportion explained to 60%. Figure 6.11 shows the performance of the model compared with actual prescribing indicators.

This simple model with four factors provides a reasonable description of prescribing behaviour and has considerable practical implications. These factors can, for example, be readily taken into account in determining prescribing budgets. Improving the predictive power of the model would be difficult because data for potential explanatory variables (for example, health status and prior use of services) are not readily available and, even if they were,

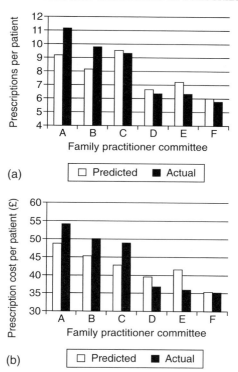

Figure 6.11   Comparison of predicted and actual prescribing indicators. The predicted costs are based on a simple regression model
Source: Data from Forster and Frost, 1991.[32]

the resultant models of prescribing behaviour might become less understandable.

Some studies have included many more variables. Healey *et al*[33] included 21 variables in a regression analysis of prescribing costs among 88 general practices in Grampian in 1990–91. Predictor variables included 10 practice and 11 patient characteristics. The regression analysis considered all potential explanatory variables of prescribing costs and made successive reductions according to various statistical criteria. This "general" to "specific" methodology may be preferable to the additive approach adopted by Forster and Frost because omitted variables can lead to problems for statistical inference.[34] The results of Healey *et al* indicate that 97% of variance in prescribing costs in Grampian can be explained by a relatively

small number of factors: list size, proportion of elderly patients, and patients living in deprived areas. Self rated health and lifestyle measures added little to the model after age and deprivation were included. The high explanatory power of the model is, however, largely attributable to the inclusion of list size as a predictor variable. As prescribing budgets are allocated by practice, it can be argued that practice, rather than patient, is the most logical unit of analysis.

An important area of analysis is prescribing costs in relation to GP fundholding. Harris and Scrivener[35] investigated whether setting of real prescribing budgets for fundholders was associated with reduction in prescribing costs, relative to non-fundholders, and how long any association lasted. The results show that prescribing costs increased by 56–59% among fundholders and by 66% among non-fundholders between 1990 and 1996 in England. Relative reduction began in the year before fundholding, was maximal in year 1, and declined in years 2 and 3 (see Fig 6.12 for the first two waves of fundholding). In subsequent years relative reduction ceased and cost of fundholders ran in parallel with continuing non-fundholders. Relative reduction appears to have been achieved by lowering average cost per items. Other studies indicate that this was probably the result of increasing generic prescribing, and possible other factors such as prescribing of less expensive items, reducing dose duration,

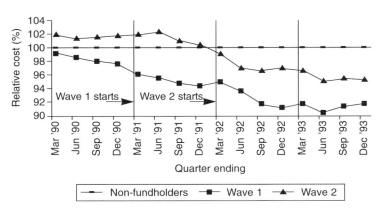

Figure 6.12 Cost per prescribing unit for first two waves of fundholding general practices in England as a percentage of the cost for the continuing non-fundholders
Source: Data from Harris and Scrivener, 1996.[35]

and lower doses. Interpretation of the results was complex because the comparative group (non-fundholders) participated in financial incentive schemes from 1993. DDDs would have been a preferable unit for analysis, but this was not possible because of the scope of the study.

Prescribing in relation to morbidity

Until recently the assumption that prescribing reflects morbidity has been hard to evaluate. For example, in the analysis reported above, Forster and Frost[32] used surrogate indices, that is, SMR, deprivation indices, and age/sex distribution. More recently, Griffiths et al[36] found that practices prescribing higher ratios of prophylaxis to bronchodilator medication had, on average, lower hospital admission rates for asthma among those aged 5–64. It is also possible, however, that the ratio may be a marker of other aspects of good asthma care. In a later study[37] they examined other variables including doctor characteristics, practice resources, prescribing, and population factors. Hospital admission rates were found to be associated with practice size (small) and night visit rates (high). Although quality of asthma prescribing was univariately associated with admissions, it did not feature in the final regression model. Several explanations were offered: high rates of night visiting could reflect higher workload, patient demand, or poorer daytime accessibility to practice. The fact that there was no association between asthma admission rates and sociodemographic variables could be the result of the approximate specification of the practice's socioeconomic profile or that, in the area being studied, socioeconomic status had a fairly uniform distribution. Furthermore, the prophylaxis/bronchodilator ratio was based on items rather than DDDs.

There have been few studies of patterns of prescribing of new drugs in general practice because routine data are usually aggregated into therapeutic groups. DDDs have been used to investigate market penetration of new drugs in relation to licensed indications in Northern Ireland.[38] DDDs were calculated for two classes of drug: angiotensin converting enzyme (ACE) inhibitors and H_2-receptor antagonists. The two indications for ACE inhibitors are managing heart failure or hypertension uncontrolled by other drugs, but they are promoted for all grades of hypertension although they are about 30 times more expensive than alternatives.

91

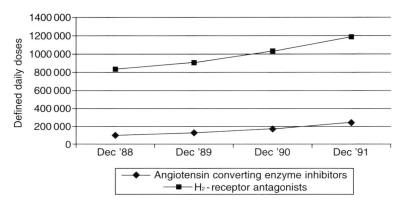

Figure 6.13 Defined daily doses in one month (December) for two drug groups in Northern Ireland
Source: Data from McGavock et al, 1993.[38]

Between 1988 and 1991 the volume of prescribing, as measured by the number of DDDs, more than doubled (Fig 6.13). Yet it is unlikely that this reflects a similar increase in the prevalence of heart failure and refractory hypertension. The increase in prescribing of H_2-receptor antagonists appears to be associated with symptomatic relief, which is more effectively managed by other drugs, than proven disease (for example, ulceration and reflux oesophagitis). As with the study by Clarke and colleagues,[19] relating DDDs to diagnoses only works for drugs with specific indications.

Qualitative issues in prescribing research

There are many aspects of prescribing that are difficult to quantify and for which routine data are not available. One key area is doctors' and patients' beliefs and attitudes towards medicines and consultations and how these relate to prescribing.

Coburn and Pit[39] investigated patients' expectations and doctors' beliefs about patient expectations when patients present with new conditions in a sample of 22 GPs and 336 of their patients in Newcastle, Australia. After controlling for presenting conditions, patients who expected medication were three times more likely to receive medication. When GPs thought that patients expected medication, however, they were 10 times more likely actually to receive medication. One implication of these findings is that practitioners prescribe more than patients expect.

Weiss et al[40] sought to relate PACT data to GPs' perception of non-clinical determinants of prescribing. From qualitative interviews with 228 GPs in southern England a questionnaire was developed to measure four areas: (1) sense of burden; (2) financial constraints and incentives; (3) prescribing as a coping strategy; and (4) patient demand. Information was also obtained on hours actually spent seeing patients. PACT data were obtained for the 228 GPs at individual and practice level. Seven measures derived from these data are shown in Box 6.2.

Box 6.2   Measures derived from PACT data: doctor, and practice characteristics

Total cost per doctor over six months divided by hours per week spent seeing patients.

Drug costs per practice population compared with Family Health Service Authority average.

Total number of prescriptions per doctor over six months divided by hours per week seeing patients.

Number of prescriptions per practice compared with the Family Health Service Authority average.

Cost per prescription for each doctor.

Proportion of generic prescriptions.

Number of antibiotic prescriptions per practice compared with Family Health Service Authority average.

Source: Weiss et al[40]

In spite of the widely held belief that there has been an increase in non-clinical prescribing, the psychosocial dimensions—(1) sense of burden, (2) prescribing as coping strategy, and (3) patient demand—were not related to any of the prescribing indicators. Only the fourth dimension relating to financial considerations was associated with prescribing; those who were concerned about adverse effects of financial pressures upon medical decisions prescribed less generically and had higher practice costs compared with the Family Health Service Authority average. These results prompt the question of whether PACT data, particularly when not specified as DDDs, are a measure of good or rational prescribing.

Avorn et al[41] investigated two drugs that controlled studies have shown not to be significantly more effective than over the counter drugs, but which were nevertheless heavily promoted as being effective (cerebral and peripheral vasodilators and propoxyphene

analgesics). Among 85 GPs in the Boston area, factors of little importance in determining prescribing decisions were advertising (68% of respondents) and patient preference (74%). In contrast, factors identified as being important were training and clinical experience (88%), and scientific papers (62%). When GPs' prescriptions were analysed, however, the results suggested that advertisements were the predominant source for beliefs about the effectiveness of these drugs.

Bradley[42] used the critical incident technique to explore the decision making processes of GPs when prescribing made them feel uncomfortable. Incidents were categorised by a panel of experts solely on the basis of the information obtained from doctors. Much prescribing, which appears irrational when judged against Parish's definition,[4] was found to come at the end of often involved processes of thought and reasoning that involved many considerations. Although Bradley suggests that doctors need education in how to avoid prescribing that is not clinically indicated, it is by no means clear, from the previously described studies, that doctors' perceptions of influences on prescribing are in fact related to their actual prescribing.

Future directions in prescribing analysis

There have been considerable advances in prescribing analysis in recent years. First, considerable work has gone into improving the analytical units: DDDs and ADQs for prescribing volumes, and ASTRO-PUs and STAR-PUs for practice populations. Second, the NHS drugs bill and the introduction of fundholding have prompted studies which have sought to identify determinants of prescribing volumes and trends. Nevertheless, the nature of prescribing data and the rapid changes in the conditions of general practice prescribing mean that the actual analysis is relatively simple in comparison to other areas of epidemiology where a greater degree of experimental control is possible.[43]

Meta-analyses

One of the main difficulties comes from the many sources of uncertainty that weaken the link between condition and treatment.[44] Although some factors such as disease prevalence and practice characteristics are predictable in theory, in practice they interact

with many determinants of prescribing such as disease definition, symptom interpretation, potential treatments, and outcome assessment. As prescribing studies usually consider a subset of these factors, interpretation of results can be daunting. One way of dealing with this situation is to refer to a meta-analysis where the methods, analyses, and results from studies on a particular topic are systematically reviewed. This is the aim of the Cochrane Library, an international network that prepares systematic reviews on the effects of health care (described in greater detail in chapter 5). Although most of the reviews are concerned with surgical, diagnostic, and drug therapy interventions, the library contains a review of the effects on patient adherence and outcomes of interventions to assist patients to follow prescriptions.[45] The collaborative review group who investigated this topic screened 1553 relevant articles. Only 13 met the strict scientific criteria of being "unconfounded randomised controlled trials of an intervention to improve adherence with prescribed medications with one or more measures of medication adherence, one or more measures of treatment outcome, at least 80% follow up of each group studies and for long-term treatments, at least six months follow up for studies with positive initial findings". Clearly criteria such as these may not be applicable to prescribing research where experimental controls are not usually possible and other approaches may have to be considered.

Bayesian inference

At present most prescribing analysis employs classic measurement inference in assessing, for example, determinants of prescribing. In many areas of medical research, an alternative methodology based on Bayes' theorem is now being used. Bayes' theorem is used to obtain the probability of a disease in a group of people with some characteristic on the basis of: (1) the overall rate of that disease (the prior probability) and (2) the likelihood of that characteristic in healthy and diseased people.[46] While the classic approach evaluates probability only on empirical observations, the bayesian approach can incorporate expert knowledge and historical observations. Bayesian analysis starts with a *prior* probability distribution derived from previous knowledge and research, and adds new data to produce a range of *posterior* probability distribution. It has been argued that conventional

statistical tests are an improper basis for policy because they tend to dichotomise results according to whether or not they are significant and therefore elicit on/off response from policy makers. In the case of a new clinical trial that shows a drug to have an adverse effect, previous knowledge about the drug is not considered in relation to the trial results. Thus, one study using conventional statistics may produce sudden changes in prescribing because the effect is statistically significant.

In contrast, bayesian statistics would indicate that the new evidence merits a shifting perception of the effects of the drug. For some clinicians and patients, this may warrant cessation of the drug while others may prefer to wait for further evidence. Lilford and Braunholz[47] argue that only the bayesian approach can address complex areas of medical research where policy decisions are required. There has been much research into prescriber and patient attitudes towards medicines, consultations, and prescribing which could be used to develop prior probabilities in relation to prescribing. Would GPs' perceptions of psychosocial determinants of prescribing, which were not found by Weiss to be statistically significant using classic inference, have elicited different findings in a bayesian analysis?

Multilevel modelling

Another challenge in prescribing research is to explain relationships between individual and aggregate level data. Multilevel modelling provides a framework within which individual level response variables can be investigated in relation to both individual and aggregate level predictors. For example, prescribing is associated with patient, doctor, and practice attributes as well as community characteristics and general social factors. One drawback of multilevel modelling is, however, the need for extensive data at the various levels. One example in prescribing research is a study by Davis and Gribben[48] of between practitioner variation in prescribing. The authors partitioned prescribing variation into that attributable to differences between patients and that resulting from differences in practitioners' propensity to prescribe. Propensity to prescribe did not decrease after controlling for individual patient and practitioner characteristics, suggesting that the level of prescribing is not associated with individual characteristics. This finding appears to support some of the

qualitative research that has highlighted the discrepancy between perceptions of psychosocial influences on prescribing and actual prescribing.

Geographical information systems

Geographical influences on prescribing were identified in the study of buccal trinitrate described earlier (see Fig 6.6). The study used a geographical information system (GIS) both to analyse and to display practice variation in prescribing. The main characteristic of a GIS is the ability to link spatially referenced data to a relational database (for example, PACT data, population data, transport routes, deprivation status). These features, together with more powerful spatial analysis tools, distinguish GIS from early mapping programs that simply displayed information (Fig 6.14).

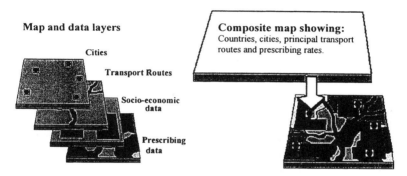

Map and data layers

Cities

Transport Routes

Socio-economic data

Prescribing data

Composite map showing:
Countries, cities, principal transport routes and prescribing rates.

Figure 6.14 Structure of a typical geographical information system
Source: Department of Medicines Management, Keele University.

Data records in GIS can be retrieved in one of two ways (Fig 6.14): first, the relational database can be searched and selections made on the basis of a feature's attributes and its values (Fig 6.15). For example, regions with higher than average levels of prescribing could be selected and then displayed. Second, GIS also allows spatial retrieval so that, for example, a map could be searched for all hospitals in urban areas. Each query could be linked to several data layers, for example, morbidity rates, prescribing rates, socioeconomic status, and transport links.

Although considerable developmental work will be required before GIS can be routinely used for prescribing analysis, the basic

Database selection

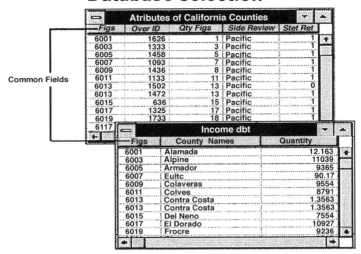

Spatial selection

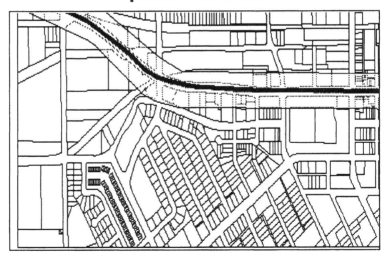

Figure 6.15   Geographical information systems—methods of data selection
Source: Department of Medicines Management, Keele University

methodology has already been used to study associations between location, environment, and disease.[49]

Prospects for prescribing analysis

One of the major resources for future prescribing analysis are databases, such as the GPRD, which contain patient prescribing and diagnostic profiles. Although the GPRD contains over 30 million years of patient histories, Jick[50] observes that it has primarily been used to investigate drug safety issues, the major impediments to more sophisticated analyses being the database's size and complexity. The GPRD could, in principle, be used to investigate prescribing in relation to patient characteristics, morbidity, and other forms of treatment. Analyses could establish whether drugs are being used for their licensed indications, what proportion of drugs is prescribed in excess of their DDDs, and what proportion of patients prescribed a given drug is subsequently referred to hospital. On the more distant horizon, electronic interchange of prescribing and dispensing records will almost certainly lead to a paradigm shift in prescribing research. The challenge over the next few years is to develop analytical tools to address the aims highlighted at the start of the chapter, namely to inform policy and to help ensure equitable distribution of resources.

1 Department of Health. *Statistics of prescriptions dispensed in the community: England 1986 to 1996*. London: Department of Health, 1997.
2 Walley T, Mantgani A. The United Kingdom general practice research database. *Lancet* 1997;**350**:1097–9.
3 Audit Commission. *A prescription for improvement. Towards more rational prescribing in general practice. Health and personal social services report, No. 1*. London: HMSO, 1994.
4 Armstrong D, Reyburn H, Jones R. A study of general practitioners' reasons for changing their prescribing behaviour. *BMJ* 1996;**312**:949–52.
5 Parish PA. Drug prescribing—the concern for all. *J R Soc Health* 1973;**4**:213–7.
6 Royal Pharmaceutical Society. *From compliance to concordance*. London: Royal Pharmaceutical Society, 1997.
7 Barber N. What constitutes good prescribing? *BMJ* 1995;**310**:923–5.
8 Harris C. Quality and measurement. In: *Prescribing in general practice* (Harris C, ed.). Oxford: Radcliffe Medical Press, 1996.
9 Law J. Who's using your data? *Medical Interface* 1997;October:45–6.
10 Ferguson J. PACT. In: *Prescribing in general practice* (Harris C, ed.). Oxford: Radcliffe Medical Press, 1996.

11 Scandinavian Simvastatin Survival Study Group.Randomised trial of cholesterol lowering in 4444 patients with coronary heart disease: the Scandinavian Simvastatin Survival Study (4S). *Lancet* 1994;**344**:1383–9.

12 Shepherd J, Cobbe SM, Ford I, Isles CG, Lorimar AR, Macfarlane P, for the West of Scotland Coronary Prevention Study Group. Prevention of coronary heart disease with pravastatin in men with hypercholesterolemia. *N Engl J Med* 1995;**333**:1301–7.

13 Edwards C, Metcalfe D, Burr A, Watson K, Steward F, Jepson M, Zwanenberg T. Influence of patient age on drug costs: an investigation to validate the prescribing unit. *Int J Pharmacy Policy* 1991;**1**:73–8.

14 Roberts SJ, Harris CM. Age, sex, and temporary resident originated prescribing units (ASTRO-PUs): new weightings for analysing prescribing of general practices in England. *BMJ* 1993;**307**:485–8.

15 Lloyd DC, Harris CM, Roberts DJ. Specific therapeutic group age-sex related prescribing units (STAR-PUs): weightings for analysing general practices' prescribing in England. *BMJ* 1995;**311**:991–4.

16 Bogle SM, Harris CM. Measuring prescribing, the shortcomings of the item. *BMJ* 1994;**308**:637–40.

17 World Health Organization. *Guideline for defined daily doses.* Oslo: WHO Collaborating Centre for Drug Statistics Methodology, 1991.

18 Prescribing Support Unit. *ADQs and STAR-PUs.* Leeds: Prescribing Support Unit, 1997.

19 Clarke K, Gray D, Hampton J. Defined daily doses: insensitive in determining disease prevalence. *Pharm J* 1994;**252**:334–5.

20 Clarke K, Gray D, Hampton J. The defined daily dose as a tool in pharmacoeconomics. *Pharmacoeconomics* 1995;**7**:280–3.

21 Hollowell J. The general practice research database: quality of morbidity data. *Population Trends* 1997;**87**:36–40.

22 McCormick A, Fleming D, Charlton J. *Morbidity statistics from general practice: fourth national study 1991-1992.* London: HMSO (Series MB5; No 3), 1995.

23 British Thoracic Society. Guidelines for the management of asthma: a summary. *BMJ* 1993;**306**:776–82.

24 Jick H, Jick S, Derby L. Validity of information recorded on general practitioner based computerised data resource in the United Kingdom. *BMJ* 1991;**302**: 766–8.

25 Jick H, Terris B, Derby L, Jick S. Further validation of information recorded on a general practitioner based computerised data resource in the United Kingdom. *Pharmacoepidemiology and Drug Safety* 1992;**1**:347–9.

26 Nazareth I, King M, Haines A, Rangel L, Myers S. Accuracy of diagnosis of psychosis on general practice computer system. *BMJ* 1993;**307**:32–4.

27 McCormick A, Fleming D, Charlton J. Who sees their general practitioner and for what reason? *Health Trends*, 1995;**27**:34–5.

28 Hinton A. Preparing for the electronic data interchange in the prescribing process. *Pharm J* 1997;**259**:767–71.

29 Paranoid about prodigy? *Pharm J* 1997;**258**:533.

30 Bateman N, Eccles M, Campbell Soutter J, Roberts SJ, Smith JM. Setting standards of prescribing performance in primary care: use of a consensus group of general practitioners and application of standards of practices in the north of England. *Br J Gen Pract* 1996;**46**:20–5.

31 Catford JC. Quality of prescribing for children in general practice. *BMJ* 1980; **280**:1435–7.

32 Forster DP, Frost CE. Use of regression analysis to explain the variation in prescribing rates and costs between family practitioner committees. *Br J Gen Pract* 1991;**41**:67–71.

33 Healey A, Yule B, Reid J. Variations in general practice prescribing costs and implications for budget setting. *Health Economics* 1994;3:47–56.
34 Stewart J. *Econometrics*. Hemel Hempstead: Phillip Allen, 1991.
35 Harris CM, Scrivener G. Fund-holding prescribing costs: the first five years. *BMJ* 1996;313:1531–4.
36 Griffiths C, Naish S, Preira S, Pereira F. Prescribing and hospital admissions for asthma in east London. *BMJ* 1996;312:418–19.
37 Griffiths C, Sturdy P, Naish J, Omar R, Dolan S, Feder G. Hospital admissions for asthma in east London: associations with characteristics of local general practitioners, prescribing, and population. *BMJ* 1997;314:482–6.
38 McGavock H, Webb CH, Johnston GD, Milligan E. Market penetration of new drugs in one United Kingdom region: implications for general practitioners and administrators. *BMJ* 1993;307:1118.
39 Coburn J, Pit S. Prescribing behaviour in clinical practice: patients' expectations and doctors' perceptions of patients' expectations—a questionnaire study. *BMJ* 1997;315:520–3.
40 Weiss MC, Fitzpatrick R, Scott DK, Goldacre MJ. Pressures on general practitioners and decisions to prescribe. *Family Practice* 1996;13:432–8.
41 Avorn J, Chen M, Hartley R. Scientific versus commercial sources of influence on the prescribing behavior of physicians. *Am J Med* 1982;73:4–8.
42 Bradley C. Factors which influence the decision whether or not to prescribe: the dilemma facing general practitioners. *Br J Gen Pract* 1992;42:454–58.
43 Hennekens CH, Buring J. *Epidemiology in medicine*. Boston: Little Brown, 1987.
44 Eddy D. Variations in physician practice: the role of uncertainty. *Health Affairs* 1983;21:75–89.
45 Haynes RB, McKibbon KA, Kanani R. *Systematic review of randomised controlled trials of the effects on patient adherence and outcomes of interventions to assist patients to follow prescriptions for medications*. Oxford: The Cochrane Library, 1996.
46 Last J. *A dictionary of epidemiology*. Oxford: Oxford University Press, 1988.
47 Lilford RJ, Braunholz D. The statistical basis of public policy: a paradigm shift is overdue. *BMJ* 1996;313:603–7.
48 Davis P, Gribben B. Rational prescribing and inter practitioner variation: a multilevel approach. *Int J Technol Assessment Health* 1995;11:428–42.
49 Barnes S, Peck A. Mapping the future of health care: GIS applications in health care analysis. *Geographic Information Systems* 1994;4:31–3.
50 Jick H. A database worth saving. *Lancet* 1997;350:1045.

7 Health economic and public health aspects of drug usage

ALAN EARL-SLATER, JEFFREY NORWOOD

Objectives

- Identify and explore economic and public health issues of drug usage.
- Illustrate the usefulness of economic modelling for resource management and health planning.
- Indicate the different types of economic assessment used to establish the economic value of drugs.
- State the factors that determine the type of assessment to use.
- Show a worked example of drug assessment.

Health economists and public health practitioners focus attention on wider aspects of health care and not just the costs and benefits of drugs themselves. They do so by taking into account wider issues surrounding the use of drugs and health:

- They establish the incidence and prevalence of disease.
- They evaluate the burden of disease and premature death on society.
- They review access to health care, equity, and quality of services.
- They consider all aspects of health including health promotion, sickness prevention, and medical and surgical services.
- They ensure that the evidence is translated into practice.

Health care is only one factor contributing to population well being. Other significant factors include: better water, drainage, and sewage systems, improved nutrition, better housing, a wider range

of goods and services available to consumers, improvements in technology, and greater personal disposable incomes.

Any public expenditure on drugs could have been used in other ways: for health promotion; other forms of treatment; better housing; training and education; or enabling more people to get back to work.

Although the total annual NHS drugs bill rises beyond £5 billion (a rise of 101% in real terms between 1980 and 1996)[12] serious questions are again being asked about the financial impact of drugs.[34] Evidence suggests that between 1989 and 1994 the shift from older to newer more expensive medicines accounted for 55% of the growth in the drugs bill.[5]

Examples of proven benefits of drugs include:

- β Blockers and diuretics can prevent stroke and coronary heart disease in hypertensive patients.
- Statins are effective in the primary and secondary prevention of acute coronary heart disease. Their targeted use has been promulgated by the Standing Medical Advisory Committee of the Department of Health.
- Angiotensin converting enzyme (ACE) inhibitors can improve longevity, reduce morbidity, and enhance the quality of life in patients with heart failure.
- Aspirin, β blockers, and statins help in secondary prevention of ischaemic heart disease.
- Eradication of *Helicobacter pylori* reduces the relapse rate of peptic ulcer disease.

Drawbacks of drugs usage include:

- Iatrogenic disease: the precipitation of diabetes with thiazide diuretics in elderly people.
- Adverse effects: an increased risk of developing breast cancer in patients taking hormone replacement therapy.
- Inappropriate use leading to loss of therapeutic efficacy: resistance to antibiotics as a result of increasing overuse and inappropriate dosage.
- Wastage of resources: the use of proton pump inhibitors for the first line symptomatic treatment of indigestion.
- Avoidance of underlying problem: symptomatic management with analgesics.

- Abuse of drugs such as flunitrazepam which has been used in date rape cases.
- Elderly patients on psychotropic drugs are more likely to fall and therefore cost the NHS additional expenses in hospital care.

Aspects to consider in assessing the clinical and economic merits of established or new drugs include:

- Establishing the impact that a particular drug has on patient's quality of life and life expectancy.
- Determining the impact that health care has on the patient's family.
- Measuring the value for money.[6–10]
- Measuring the additional costs involved in managing patients on particular drugs (screening, testing, monitoring, and dealing with side effects).
- Identifying the impact that drugs have on other aspects of health care such as hospitalisation rates, residential, and nursing home care costs.
- Effects on local authorities or social services.

In December 1997 the UK Government announced plans to set up a National Institute for Clinical Excellence (NICE) to establish the clinical and economic merits of drugs. Until this Institute is working there is no national assessment system to measure the clinical or economic merits of drugs, despite the fact that revenue spend has always taken the larger part of all NHS health care spend.[13] This can be contrasted with the long standing system to demonstrate a structured approach to assessing capital investment in the NHS.

Alternative perspectives

Although it is important to look at the broader economic aspects of health care interventions, individual decisions are usually made on their individual merits and from a particular perspective. A doctor may not care so much about costs that fall outside her budget. Drugs that allow patients to be cared for in their home rather than in residential care may add extra burdens on the local social service budgets. Drugs that get people out of hospital earlier can put additional pressures on the primary health care, social service, and local authority budgets. These budgetary problems

can be reduced if joint budgets or virement exists between health and social service authorities.[8] It is easier to acknowledge different perspectives than to reconcile them. Yet reconciling the different perspectives is one of the major tasks faced by decision makers in health care.

Background

When a new drug comes on the market we do not know much about it. There will be evidence about the product's safety, efficacy, and quality (three hurdles) from the clinical trial data and submissions to the licensing authorities. But there is a lot we do not know.[8-10] The clinical trial data are not generally available from the companies or licensing authorities. There is also uncertainty about how best to incorporate the drug into the clinical and financial environments in the NHS. Patient compliance, optimum doses, use in patients with concomitant disease, and the longer term effects of the drug are unknown.

There is no requirement to prove that the drug is better than another already on the market or that the drug is actually worth buying: a fourth hurdle.

"Is it worth it?" is a question that continues to be raised in health policy. It is neither new nor unique to the UK. In late 1997 the World Health Organization called for a fourth hurdle to be established.[11] Although the WHO call has been echoed by others, the methods of determining value for money of drugs are fraught with practical and methodological difficulties.[6-10] For example, we do not know all of the therapeutic or clinical merits of any drug until it has been put into practice.[8] A few examples illustrate this point. Amantadine was originally used as an antiviral agent but has now been found to have clinical merit in patients with Parkinson's disease. Calcitonin, originally used for Paget's disease of the bone, has, through clinical experience, clinical merit in the management of postmenopausal osteoporosis. Penicillamine, originally used for patients with Wilson's disease, now has a role to play in patients with rheumatoid arthritis. The classic example is thalidomide that was initially used as an anti-morning sickness product in the late 1950s and early 1960s, and associated with serious fetal deformities. The product has recently been seen to have a positive therapeutic role for patients with AIDS, Behçet's disease, and leprosy. If a

fourth hurdle is used at the early stages of a drug's market life this may abrogate opportunities for determining its true merits.

A drug that starts off being poor value for money may, through clinical experience, turn out to be good value. The difference between using epoetin in practice compared with the clinical trial setting was that lower doses were required and fewer blood transfusions were necessary. The economic and clinical merits of drugs need to be constantly reviewed.[8 10]

When sufficient data are available, Table 7.1 can be used to decide if a drug is good value for money.

Table 7.1   This drug regimen compared with the alternative use of resources

	Costs less	Costs the same	Costs more
Fewer benefits	4	7	9
Same benefits	2	5	8
Greater benefits	1	3	6

The best drugs are those that are in cell 1: they cost less than the alternative use of resources and provide greater benefits. The least desirable drugs are those in cell 9: the drug costs more but provides fewer benefits.

Costs

Costs can be classified according to where they fall:[8]

- Direct costs: clinical examination, drug acquisition, laboratory, health professionals, community care, residential care, local authority, or social services.
- Indirect costs: incurred by the patient and their family in travelling to the health care facility; the monetary value of the wages the patient loses through being off sick, or the family's caring costs in looking after the patient.
- Intangible costs: the personal pain and grief, the loss of leisure or pleasure from life as a result of the disease or treatment regimen.

There are various forms of cost:[6–8]

- Total costs: the aggregate figure of all costs involved.
- Average costs: total costs divided by volume of activity.

- Marginal cost: the change in total costs if one more patient is treated with the intervention.
- Fixed costs: these do not change with activity levels (rent, heating, lighting, and minimum staff expenditures).
- Variable costs: depend on the number of patients treated (the drugs bill, administration, diagnosis).
- Opportunity cost: the value of benefits that would have been achieved if the next best option was taken. For example, health authorities and prescribers were urged to follow the evidence supporting the use of lipid lowering drugs, statins, in secondary prevention of heart disease. Estimated costs in treating all patients in the West Midlands (10% of the UK population) for secondary prevention would be £15.1 million in the 1997–98 financial year. This money could be spent on intensive health promotion campaigns to discourage smoking—a primary cause of heart disease. The opportunity cost of prescribing statins for secondary prevention is the value of the benefits that would have come from the intensive health promotion campaigns.

If health care data are not available for the UK setting, then evidence from other countries may be considered, subject to two reservations:[8 12]

- Data are usually pulled out of context.
- The range of costs can vary widely.

Evidence from a recent international review of the use of misoprostol for prophylaxis against gastric ulcers induced by non-steroidal anti-inflammatory drugs illustrates the point:[12]

- Ambulatory care costs ranged from $US256 in France to $US901 in the USA.
- Drug acquisition costs for three months on misoprostol 800 µg/day ranged from $US129 in France to $US180 in the USA.
- The duration of hospital stays ranged from seven days in the USA to 18 days in Belgium.
- Total direct health care costs for a medical patient ranged from $US1548 in the UK to $US3450 in the USA.
- Total direct health care costs for surgical patients ranged from $US2533 in the UK to $US15 700 in the USA.

Outcomes

The purpose of any health care intervention is to have a positive impact on the patient's health status or life expectancy. Attention must therefore be drawn to the outcomes of interventions.[13] At this stage two sources of data can be considered: phase III clinical trials or data from other countries. There is no mandatory requirement in the UK that any data from the trials are made available. As with costs, the main difficulty with using outcome data from other countries is that they may be out of context.

Two aspects of health outcome measures to consider are the type of instrument used and the data returned.[8]

Generic instruments

These are applicable in a variety of diseases and at different levels of one disease. An example includes the uniform index of activities of daily living (ADL).

Specific instruments

These are applicable only in certain diseases and at certain levels of the disease. The Alzheimer's Disease Assessment Scale (ADAS) is an example.

Health index

This is a single number representing the health status of the patient. An example is the index of health related quality of life (IHQOL) which measures social, psychological, and physical aspects of health status and returns a single number that is said to represent the status of the person.

Health profile

This is a collection of numbers representing the health status of the patient. An example is the Sickness Impact Profile (SIP) which contains 12 categories covering how the sickness relates to their recreation, work, emotions, home life, sleep, rest, eating, mobility, communication, ambulation, and social interaction.

The advantage of using more than one health status measurement instrument is that a wider picture of the patient's health status may be identified.[8 13] The disadvantage is that, with so many instruments

being used, and many others that could have been used, it is difficult to summarise the impact of the intervention.

When multiple outcomes arise,[8 13] one can:

- Decide in advance the most clinically significant outcome
- Convert the outcomes into money terms
- Convert the outcomes into units of utility (for example, a quality adjusted life year or QALY—see below).

Converting outcomes into money terms has been attempted using methods such as willingness to pay.[6-9] Two issues in willingness to pay are (1) willingness to pay may be intrinsically related to ability to pay, and (2) who to ask.

One measure of utility is the quality adjusted life year (QALY) which seeks to capture the change in quality of life and the change in life expectancy from a health care intervention. For example, if a new drug improves a patient's life expectancy by three years and allows him or her to live with a quality of life denoted as 0.6 (with 0 being death and 1 being perfect health), then it would be expected that the drug allows the patient to have 1.8 QALYs. The main debates with QALYs are whether:[6-10]

- QALYs can be compared over time or across different patients.
- A naturally lower life expectancy, for example, of elderly people, implies that the QALY is biased against them.
- Only the patient's QALY matters.
- QALY results are dependent on how the quality of life (QoL) aspect is captured. Use of different instruments can lead to different conclusions.

Discounting

In normal practice the costs and benefits from any particular health care intervention will be spread over time. Today's value of these future costs and benefits can be established in principle by discounting. As the costs and benefits of a hepatitis A virus immunisation programme were expected to accrue over time, one analysis has discounted them at a rate of 6%.[14] This means that the future benefits of the immunisation programme are considered at today's value, as are the future costs. Different discount rates can be used to reflect the speed with which the value of the costs or benefits are expected to change over time.[6 8 9] Two main issues

to consider in discounting are (1) what discount rate(s) to use, and (2) whether or not costs are discounted at the same rate(s) as benefits.

Sensitivity analysis

Sensitivity analysis is a technique of establishing how responsive study results are to changes in the underlying data or set of assumptions. Sensitivity analysis has three uses:

- To reflect the influence of uncertainty.
- To allow local data to be put into the analysis.
- To review different possible scenarios without inconveniencing patients or health care staff.

What kind of economic assessment can be used?

Figure 7.1 shows different types of economic assessment that can be used on drugs.[8] There are two key questions in the decision

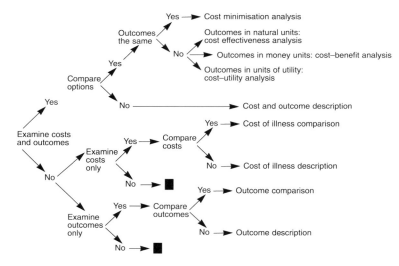

Figure 7.1   Economic Assessment Decision Tree
Source: Alan Earl-Slater, Department of Medicines Management, Keele University.

tree: (1) Are costs and outcomes considered? (2) Are different treatment regimens considered?

The decision tree has a variety of uses:[8]

- It reveals the similarities and differences of each type of assessment.
- It acts as a checklist to determine what type of assessment was performed compared with what someone claims to have performed.
- It shows what has to be covered in each type of assessment.
- It helps identify the main types of assessment that can be used in establishing the merits of new drugs.

Reading the decision tree from left to right, one can establish what has to be done to achieve a particular assessment. For example, if only the costs of a drug are determined and we do not compare it with anything else, then this is a cost description. If costs and outcomes of a particular drug are considered, then this is a cost and outcome description.

Let us suppose that the UK's new National Institute of Clinical Effectiveness claims that it has carried out a cost effectiveness analysis. Then reading the decision tree from right to left the key aspects of cost effectiveness analysis can be established: (1) the costs and outcomes of more than one treatment regimen are considered; and (2) outcomes are in natural units.

Costs and outcomes of different treatment regimens

There are four types of economic assessment which capture costs and benefits of different treatment regimens. They differ in how they measure outcomes.

Cost minimisation

This occurs where outcomes from different treatment regimens are found to be, or can safely be assumed to be, the same or not significantly different. Salewski et al[15] used cost minimisation analysis of sequential treatment with ofloxacin or ciprofloxacin in hospitalised patients.

Cost effectiveness

Outcomes are in natural units and are found to differ in magnitude or distribution depending on what option is considered. Examples include cognitive function, lumbar flexion, cholesterol level, symptom free days, systolic blood pressure, wound infection

healing rates, and visual acuity. Magid *et al*[16] established the cost effectiveness of doxycycline therapy compared with single dose azithromycin therapy in women with uncomplicated cervical *Chlamydia trachomatis* infection. The outcomes measured were the number of major and minor sequelae of *Chlamydia trachomatis*.

Cost–benefit

Outcomes are transformed into monetary values. Ginsberg and Lev[17] performed a cost–benefit analysis of riluzole for the treatment of amyotrophic lateral sclerosis.

Cost–utility

Outcomes are transformed into units of utility or satisfaction (for example, a QALY). Kennedy *et al*[18] performed a cost–utility analysis of chemotherapy and best supportive care in non-small cell lung cancer.

What factors determine the type of analysis undertaken?

The four key points are:

- The question one wants answered
- The availability of data
- The length of time one has to do the analysis
- How soon one needs the results.

What calculations can be made on the data?

There is no one correct method of calculation.[6–10 12] Each approach offers a different insight into the resource implications of options available.

Total costs and benefits

This will show whether or not the costs can be absorbed in budgets.

Average costs and benefits

Averages can be distorted by a few extreme numbers and may be misleading because of the distribution of data (for example, if it is heavily skewed).

Marginal analysis of costs and benefits

The change in costs and the change in benefits are useful if the decisions are to be made on slightly more or slightly less of a particular activity.

Economic elements of Alzheimer's disease and donepezil: a worked example

The purpose of modelling the potential impact of a drug is:[8][19]

- To help decision makers make informed choices.
- To enhance the understanding of practical issues and resource implications surrounding the drug.
- To share ideas and knowledge of the issues involved with a wider audience.
- To provoke discussion.
- To provide a platform for wider and deeper debate.

Burden of disease

From an estimated 600 000 people with dementia in the UK, an estimated 400 000 have Alzheimer's disease. This disease can be categorised as mild, moderate, or severe, but no epidemiological evidence is routinely available on how many patients are in each group. What is known is that the incidence and prevalence of Alzheimer's disease increase with age: 5% of those aged 65–74, 10% of those aged 75–84, and 30–40% of those aged 85 years or older are considered to have Alzheimer's disease.

Costs

Direct costs

As Table 7.2 shows the direct costs currently associated with Alzheimer's disease in the UK include current medication, inpatient and outpatient costs, community care, and residential and nursing home stays. Current medication includes antipsychotics, hypnotics, antidepressants, and anxiolytics. Direct costs also arise in other sectors of society: £9.5 million in local authority and social services budgets. Although direct costs are also incurred in the private

113

Table 7.2   Direct costs currently associated with Alzheimer's disease in the UK

	Costs (£ million)
Direct costs to the NHS	
Current medication	290
	(antipsychotics, hypnotics, antidepressants, anxiolytics)
Hospital inpatient stays ⎫	262
Hospital outpatient visits ⎭	
General practice	4
Community care	No evidence
Other health professionals	No evidence
Residential care and nursing homes	678
Direct costs of the disease to other sectors in society	
Local authority	30
Social services	65
Private sector	No evidence

Source: Midland Therapeutic Review and Advisory Committee report on donepezil 1997, Keele University, Department of Medicines Management.

sector, no data are available on its magnitude. Total direct costs are currently £1329 million per year.

Drug acquisition costs

Table 7.3 shows the other costs associated with donepezil. Accurate diagnosis involves individual assessment and the use of computer tomography (CT) scanning. Assessment by psychiatric community nurses is nominally set at £10 per patient and assessment by a consultant is £25 per patient. One CT scan costs between £110 and £175 per patient.

Indirect costs

Informal care costs, estimated to lie between £12 000 and £33 000 per patient family, imply costs of between £4.8 billion and £13.2 billion per year for the country. Lost productivity of the patient, proxied as the lost earnings of the patient by not working, lowering their job commitments, or dying prematurely, is estimated to be £0.3 million per annum.

Table 7.3   Direct costs associated with donepezil

	Per patient per 28 days (£)	Per patient per year (£)	For all UK patients for 1 year (£ million)
Drug acquisition costs			
5 mg	68.32	890	356
10 mg	95.76	1250	500
Costs as a result of side effects			
Hospitalisation	No evidence		
Non-hospitalisation			
Costs of diagnosis and management			
Doctor	15 per visit		
Psychiatric community nurse	10 per assessment		
Consultant	25 per assessment		
CT scan including interpretation	110–175 per scan		

Outcomes

The main published evidence on the efficacy of donepezil relates to a 12 week, multicentre, double blind, placebo controlled trial.[20] Patients were randomised to receive placebo (40 patients), 1 mg donepezil per day (42 patients), 3 mg donepezil per day (40 patients), or 5 mg donepezil per day (39 patients). The patients in the trial were aged between 55 and 85 and had been diagnosed with mild to moderate Alzheimer's disease one year before the start of the trial. The patients also had to have a *reliable caregiver*, although it is not clear what is meant by the term. Of the patients 12% failed to complete the study.[20]

Various outcome measures were used in the trials. The Alzheimer's Disease Assessment Scale—cognitive subscore (ADAS-cog) examines selected aspects of cognitive performance such as memory, orientation, attention, reasoning, language, and praxis. The score runs from 0 to 70 with higher scores indicating greater cognitive impairment. Without any treatment patients with mild to moderate Alzheimer's disease have an estimated 6–12 unit reduction in cognitive score.

Other instruments used in the trials include: the Clinical Global Impression of Change (CGIC); the uniform activities of daily living scale (ADL); the Mini Mental State Examination (MMSE); the Clinical Dementia Rating (CDR); the patient's quality of life scores as assessed by the patient (QoL-P); and the patient's quality of life scores as assessed by the caregiver (QoL-C).[20]

Compared with the baseline measures, the adjusted average ADAS-cog score was reduced by 2.5 units in the 5 mg group compared with placebo, and down by 1.4 units in the 3 mg arm of the trial. These results were found to be statistically significant. No significant changes were found in any other measures used in this trial.

Even if the results are statistically significant, are they clinically significant? In practical terms, do patients or health care professionals notice any effect? Health care professionals have argued that a 4 unit change in ADAS-cog score is the minimum change considered clinically significant.[21] Put slightly differently, although the results of the clinical trials show statistical significance on one aspect of health (cognitive function), the results are not clinically significant.

Despite using some of the most useful outcome measurement instruments available,[8 13 20] the trial on donepezil[20] failed to find clinically significant results from intervention. This result will not stop patients or their families demanding the drug.

Costs and outcomes

As indicated earlier, sensitivity analysis allows one to explore the robustness of results to changes in the underlying variables. The following analysis uses direct costs as seen in Table 7.3, and the clinical trial result of an ADAS-cog score reduction from baseline of 2.5 units for patients on 5 mg donepezil.

Table 7.4 provides an indication of the costs associated with different possible medicines management scenarios. The first column of figures gives the direct costs of each scenario. The second column shows how much it would cost to achieve an average 2.5 unit reduction in ADAS-cog scores for each patient receiving the drug. The costs range from £935 to over £3620 per patient receiving the drug.

Table 7.4   Costs associated with different scenarios for the treatment of Alzheimer's disease

UK treatment alternatives	Direct costs for the scenario (£ million)	Annual average cost to achieve 2.5 unit reduction in cognition impairment per patient (£)
Scenario A: 400 000 patients with Alzheimer's disease go to their GPs, and all receive the drug for one year. No consultant referral and no scanning	374	935
Scenario B: 600 000 patients with dementia (including 400 000 with Alzheimer's disease) go to their GPs and all receive the drug for one year. No consultant referral and no scanning	561	935
Scenario C:. GPs send all 400 000 patients with Alzheimer's disease to a specialist consultant and for a CT scan. Assume 50% receive the drug for one year	244	1220
Scenario D: GPs send 10% of the 400 000 patients to the consultant and then for a CT scan. Assume all these patients receive the drug for one year	48.8	1205
Scenario E: GPs send all 400 000 patients for cognitive assessment by a community nurse and then for a CT scan. Assume half receive the drug for one year	238	1190
Scenario F: GPs send 10% of the 400 000 patients for cognitive assessment by a community nurse and then a CT scan. Assume 10% of these patients subsequently receive the drug for one year	14.5	3620
Scenario G: assume 5% (464 000) of total UK population aged 65 and over are referred to a consultant and receive a CT scan. Half have mild to moderate Alzheimer's disease and receive the drug for one year	283	1220
Scenario H: based on the evidence of Alzheimer's disease by age group assume that: • 5% of 65–74 year olds (252 500) • 10% of 75–84 year olds (314 000) • 30% of 85 + year olds (327 000) are referred to a consultant and receive a CT scan. Assume half subsequently receive the drug for one year	545	1220

Note: It is assumed that the general practitioner sees each patient who receives the drug at the start, six months in to and at the end of the treatment year.

117

Efficacy or effectiveness?

The change in cognitive function was found under heavily controlled clinical trial conditions.[20] It is doubtful if these outcomes would be achieved in a more natural setting, that is, in practice.

This raises an issue concerning the difference between efficacy and efficiency:

- Efficacy: is the degree to which a health care intervention does what it is intended to do under ideal conditions (for example, as in clinical trials).
- Effectiveness: is what a health care intervention achieves in practice (that is, in natural settings).

Benchmarking

Economic modelling helps set out a platform upon which subsequent new drugs can be compared. Donepezil is the first drug in a new class of drugs aiming to treat Alzheimer's disease, and although the benefits are small the costs are large. Subsequent data should be compared with the benchmarks provided in this chapter.

Conclusions

- There will never be enough resources to satisfy all demands on health care.
- Choices have to be made.
- Every choice entails a sacrifice (an opportunity cost).
- A collection of costs and outcomes can be identified and used in analysis.
- The robustness of results needs examination (sensitivity analysis).
- The economic and clinical merits of drugs need to be constantly reviewed.
- Modelling costs and outcomes provide a benchmark for future drugs.
- Health economics is an important aid to decision making.

Further reading

Bishop M, Kay J, Mayer C. *The regulatory challenge*. Oxford: Oxford University Press, 1995.

Bowling A. *Research methods in health*. Milton Keynes: Open University Press, 1997.

Davis P. *Managing medicines: public policy and therapeutic drugs*. Milton Keynes: Open University Press, 1997.

Dixon M, Murray T, Jenner D. *The locality commissioning handbook*. Oxford: Radcliffe Medical Press, 1997.

Glynn JJ, Perkins DA, Stewart S. *Achieving value for money*. London: WB Saunders Co, 1996.

Helms RB (ed). *Competitive strategies in the pharmaceutical industry*. Washington DC: The AEI Press, 1996.

Jackson P, Lavender M (eds). *Public services yearbook 1996–9*. London: Pitman Publishing, 1997.

Marinker M (ed). *Controversies in health care policies*. London: BMJ Publishing Group, 1994.

Riley C, Warner M, Pullen A, Piggot CS. *Releasing resources to achieve health gain*. Oxford: Radcliffe Medical Press, 1995.

Sanderson D, Brown J. *Managing medicine: a survival guide*. London: FT Healthcare, 1997.

Tushman ML, Anderson P. *Managing strategic innovation and change*. Oxford: Oxford University Press, 1997.

Wilson J (ed). *Integrated care management: the path to success?* Oxford: Butterworth Heinemann, 1997.

1 Office of Health Economics. *Compendium of health statistics*, 10th edn. London: Office of Health Economics, 1997.

2 Office of National Statistics. *Economic trends*. London: Office of National Statistics, 1997.

3 Earl-Slater A, Bradley C. The inexorable rise in the National Health Service drugs bill: recent policies, future prospects. *Public Administration: An International Quarterly* 1996;**74**:393–411.

4 Dent THS, Hawke S. Too soon to market: doctors and patients need more information before drugs enter routine use. *BMJ* 1997;**315**:1248–9.

5 Marchant N. *Drivers of the growth in medicines expenditure*. London: Office of Health Economics, 1997.

6 Bootman JL, Townsend RJ, McGhan WF. *Principles of pharmacoeconomics*, 2nd edn. Cincinnati Ohio: W Harvey Whitney Books Co, 1996.

7 Drummond MF, O'Brien BJ, Stoddart GL, Torrance G. *Methods for the economic evaluation of health care programmes*, 2nd edn. Oxford: Oxford University Press, 1997.

8 Earl-Slater A, Mucklow JC, Bashford JNR, Green JRB. How to apply pharmacoeconomic principles to local settings. *Dis Manage Health Outcomes* 1997;**2**:65–76.

9 Sloan FA (ed.) *Valuing health care*. Cambridge: Cambridge University Press, 1996.

10 Sloan FA, Grabowski HG. The impact of cost-effectiveness on public and private policies in health care: an international perspective. *Soc Sci Med* 1997;**45**:507–647.

11 World Health Organization. *Health for all for the twenty-first century—the health policy for Europe.* Denmark: WHO's European Regional Committee, 1997.

12 Mason J. The generalisability of pharmacoeconomic studies. *Pharmacoeconomics* 1997;**11**:503–14.

13 Bowling A. *Measuring health*, 2nd edn. Milton Keynes: Open University Press, 1997.

14 Arnal JM, Frisas O, Garuz R, Antonanzas F. Cost effectiveness of hepatitis A virus immunisation in Spain. *Pharmacoeconomics* 1997;**2**:361–73.

15 Salewski E, Bassaris HP, Calangu S, Kitzes R, Kosmidis J, Raz R, Kompan L. Cost-minimisation analysis of sequential treatment with ofloxacin or ciprofloxacin in hospitalised patients. *Pharmacoeconomics* 1997;**11**:359–66.

16 Magid D, Douglas JM Jr, Schwartz JS. Doxycycline compared with azithromycin for treating women with genital *Chlamydia trachomatis* infections: an incremental cost-effectiveness analysis. *Ann Intern Med* 1996;**124**:389–99.

17 Ginsberg GM, Lev B. Cost–benefit analysis of riluzole for the treatment of amyotrophic lateral sclerosis. *Pharmacoeconomics* 1997;**12**:578–84.

18 Kennedy W, Reinharz D, Tessier G, Contandriopoulos A-P, Trabut I, Champagne F, Ayoub J. Cost–utility analysis of chemotherapy and best supportive care in non-small cell lung cancer. *Pharmacoeconomics* 1995;**8**:316–23.

19 Buxton MJ, Drummond MF, van Hout BA, Prince RL, Sheldon TA, Szucs T, Vray M. Modelling in economic evaluation: an unavoidable fact of life. *Health Economics* 1997;**6**:217–27.

20 Rogers SL, Friedhoff LT, and the Donepezil Study Group. The efficacy and safety of donepezil in patients with Alzheimer's disease. Results of a US multicentre, randomised, placebo-controlled trial. *Dementia* 1996;**7**:293–303.

21 Pharmacy Practice Division of the Common Services Agency for the Scottish Health Service. *Evaluated information on donepezil March 13 1997.* Edinburgh: Common Services Agency, Scottish Health Service, 1997.

8 National structures to facilitate good medicines management

TOM WALLEY

Objectives

- To identify and describe the organisations which may contribute to good management of medicines within the UK.
- To facilitate the access of the reader to these organisations.

There are several organisations with responsibilities for enhancing the management of medicines at a national level in the UK; this chapter aims to describe some of them. Some are mainly managerial (for example, NHS Executive Prescribing Branch, Prescription Pricing Authority [PPA]), and some mainly professional/academic (NHS Centre for Reviews and Dissemination, UK Cochrane Centre). There is some overlap between these categories. All of the organisations described here are funded by the taxpayer, some directly through the NHS (for example, the Centre for Reviews and Dissemination, the National Prescribing Centre) and some by local NHS (Development and Evaluation Committee) or indirectly by the Department of Health (Drug and Therapeutics Bulletin). Some of the organisations are statutory, that is, they exist by virtue of legislation (for example, Medicines Control Agency, European Medicines Evaluation Agency, PPA), but most are not.

Some of these organisations, particularly the managerial or statutory ones, focus almost exclusively on drug use (PPA, National Prescribing Centre). Others, particularly the professional and academic ones, have arisen from the current impetus for evidence

based medicine and enhancing clinical effectiveness and efficiency, and only consider medicines use alongside many other NHS interventions for patients. This is important, because it must be recognised that looking at medicines alone is not adequate in considering the overall management of patients within the NHS or in considering how the NHS deploys resources.

These organisations have largely developed over many years without clear coordination or an overall NHS prescribing support plan. Although they generally cooperate well with one another, there is some duplication of effort.

The latest White Paper[1] will further alter the context of prescribing within the NHS, unifying prescribing budgets and cash limiting drug budgets within the Primary Care Groups or Trusts; this will alter the needs of prescribers and commissioners for information and we are likely as a result to see changes in how these organisations work in the future.

Statutory agencies

The Medicines Control Agency (MCA) is charged with safeguarding public health by ensuring that all medicines on the UK market meet appropriate standards of safety, quality, and efficacy. It does this through the initial licensing of medicines in the UK, and by monitoring the safety of medicines after the licence has been granted. It provides information on drug hazards and ways of improving the safe use of medicines through its quarterly bulletins *Current Problems in Pharmacovigilance* and links with the *British National Formulary*. The MCA is guided in its work by its expert professional committees, of which the most important is the Committee on Safety of Medicines. It is this Committee that ultimately recommends licensing or withdrawal of a licence. The criteria for the licensing of drugs (safety, quality, and efficacy) are governed by the Medicines Act 1968, which at the time was revolutionary. It might, however, be criticised in the 1990s as inadequate, because it prevents consideration of the relative effectiveness or cost effectiveness of medicines in the UK as part of the licensing procedure.

A new European system for the authorisation of medicines came into effect in January 1995, managed by the London based European Medicines Evaluation Agency (EMEA). This coordinates the various resources of the national licensing

authorities and allows two licensing procedures: the centralised, whereby products are considered directly by the central body after consultation (obligatory for all biotechnology products), and the decentralised, whereby a drug licence issued in one country of the European Union is recognised by the other countries after some consultation. The EMEA now takes on many of the roles of the national bodies, although obviously not totally superseding them.

The Prescription Pricing Authority is a special health authority with two main functions: to ensure payment of community pharmacists and dispensing doctors for the dispensing of NHS prescriptions, and to provide prescribing and dispensing information from primary care to the NHS (to prescribers, health authorities, and the Department of Health)—PACT (Prescribing Analysis and Cost) data, discussed more fully in chapter 6. These data are an important resource for prescribers and for health authority prescribing advisers in trying to manage medicines and medicine budgets.

The PPA has other roles: it also manages the NHS low income scheme and is responsible for the prevention of prescribing and dispensing fraud within the NHS. It publishes commentaries on topical and important aspects of prescribing, as a centrefold within the quarterly PACT returns to GPs. More recently, it has started to produce data on prescribing by nurses: some nurses have recently been granted limited prescribing rights within a special formulary—those nurses with a district nurse or health visitor qualification, who have completed a nurse prescriber's training course and who are employed by an NHS Trust or a general practice.

Managerial agencies

Within the NHS Executive is a Pharmacy and Prescribing Branch, which has responsibilities for implementing Government policy related to prescribing and for the management of prescribing in England, particularly in primary care. The Scottish, Welsh and Northern Ireland Offices have similar branches. Working within the branch are civil servants, including former health care professionals and managers. The Pharmacy and Prescribing Branch issues Executive Letters (ELs) to the NHS through the NHS Executive on a range of important issues related to prescribing. Every year it issues guidance on how to

set practice prescribing budgets to the health authority prescribing advisers (for example, EL 97/63), but it also provides advice on other issues such as prescribing at the interface between primary and secondary care (EL 91/127), the prescribing of high cost drugs (for example, EL 95/5 and EL 95/97), and managing the introduction of new drugs (EL 94/72), as well as providing directives on a range of other related issues. Although most ELs are not strictly legally binding, they set the framework within which health authorities manage prescribing. The Pharmacy and Prescribing Branch also provides advice to the rest of the Department of Health and to the Secretary of State for Health on issues related to medicines use and expenditure, including the implications of other Government policies for prescribing and vice versa. The Pharmacy and Prescribing Branch is supported by the Prescribing Support Unit, a unit in Leeds funded directly by the NHS Executive, which assists in the analysis of prescribing data and which undertakes development of tools to further both the management and the academic understanding of prescribing.

The Pharmacy and Prescribing Branch has also been instrumental in promoting the development of the computer decision support system for prescribing currently under test in PRODIGY (see chapter 9).

Other branches within the Department of Health have responsibilities for medicines pricing and for monitoring the profitability of the pharmaceutical industry in the UK (see chapter 4).

The National Prescribing Centre based in Liverpool is a new health service body funded directly by the NHS Executive and has a number of major roles around facilitating high quality prescribing:

1   To provide training and education, mainly for prescribing advisers in health authorities in their role to improve prescribing and medicines use, but also to GPs (partly direct and partly through GP trainers) and to a wider professional and managerial audience, in order to improve further their knowledge of, and approach to, prescribing issues. As part of this, the National Prescribing Centre publishes the monthly *MeReC Bulletin*, a medicines information bulletin sent to GPs throughout England, and a range of other materials.

2   Information: to help coordinate the provision of information on medicines and prescribing related issues and clinical effectiveness to health authorities, their advisers, and GPs, and to help inform national policy on these issues.

3   To help publicise the many good regional and local initiatives to enhance prescribing which are currently under way.

The National Prescribing Centre was formed in 1996 from units established by the NHS Executive to support the Indicative Prescribing Scheme and other prescribing initiatives and, although it retains some of the functions of these units, it now works to a wider agenda recognising the emphasis on evidence based health care, the move towards a primary care led NHS and local commissioning, and other developments in policy and technology within the NHS. Its focus traditionally has been on prescribing in primary care, but with the increased move towards disease management across the primary care/secondary care interface and the merging of prescribing budgets across primary and secondary care, its work is now increasing in these areas.

NHS research and development and professional/ academic organisations

The NHS has a strategy for research and development, which is aimed at creating a "knowledge based health service in which clinical, managerial, and policy decisions are based on sound information and scientific developments". This strategy depends heavily on the creation and careful evaluation of evidence of clinical effectiveness and cost effectiveness, and then on the implementation of this evidence in practice. The practicalities and difficulties of achieving this are discussed more fully in chapters 4 and 5. This strategy has funded a number of national and local bodies charged with the production and review of evidence, and the promotion of evidence based practice.

Several arms of NHS research and development strategy may influence prescribing. These include the Health Technology Assessment Programme, the Information Systems Strategies and the professional/academic organisations created as a result, and directly funded research into aspects of prescribing.

Health Technology Assessment

Health Technology Assessment (HTA) is defined as an assessment of the clinical, social, ethical, and financial impact of new technologies (including medicines), aiming to evaluate such technologies before they become established in clinical practice. It aims to provide the information to allow an informed choice for clinicians, managers, and others as to whether a new technology should become used within the NHS and to what extent. The need for this kind of assessment is clear: new technologies often enter clinical practice without adequate evaluation, with the result that technologies of poor effectiveness or poor cost effectiveness may gain a foothold within practice, or conversely that other effective and cost effective technologies may be underused (for example anti-platelet therapy in cardiovascular disease), because either their clinical benefits are not recognised or they are considered too expensive. In many ways, medicines are relatively favoured under the HTA process, because they have extensive evidence of clinical efficacy, which is required for licensing purposes, before the drug is ever launched. This contrasts starkly with the relative lack of evidence for many other technologies. The criteria for medicine licensing (efficacy, safety, and quality) are not, however, necessarily adequate for prescribing, where the criteria should be effectiveness and cost effectiveness as well as safety. Effectiveness here means *the extent and likelihood of desired clinical effects on the patient* in comparison to that achieved by other treatments. Clearly the evidence underpinning this broad definition of effectiveness may be weak when a drug is first marketed, and the drug will require further evaluation before its widespread use in the NHS can be recommended. HTA aims to provide this evaluation.

The first results of the HTA of pharmaceuticals should be published in 1998. Problems with the process include its relatively slow speed of reaction, in part because of the rigour of the evaluations: the use of drugs disseminates far more rapidly than that of other technologies, and the speed of the assessment process becomes crucial. In recognition of this, a process of *fast tracking* of particularly urgent topics exists within the programme, whereby topics can be dealt with more rapidly. HTA cannot address all new drugs and must prioritise. It is also important to appreciate that it is not a once and for all assessment: as with drug safety, it is an

iterative process so as new information about a drug or other technology becomes available, an assessment needs to be reconsidered. Despite these difficulties, HTA has the potential to reform the way in which we evaluate new drugs for use within the NHS.

HTA is managed by the National Co-ordinating Centre for Health Technology Assessment in Southampton.

NHS R&D Information Systems Strategy

This strategy aims to provide the information to allow the implementation of more effective health care. It funds two main national bodies,[2] but its aims are also supported by many local bodies. Given the importance of prescribing as a health care intervention, the work of these centres will inevitably include reviews, which will greatly help to define what the most appropriate use of medicines is in many conditions. (Reasons why this evidence based approach is not entirely adequate are considered in chapters 5 and 6).

The UK Cochrane Centre (UKCC) based in Oxford aims to facilitate and coordinate the preparation and maintenance of systematic reviews of evidence on issues related to health care, and to ensure their dissemination, so as to help health professionals, managers, and patients make informed decisions about health care. It is part of the international Cochrane Collaboration which has similar aims, and supports researchers within the UK who are contributing to the Collaboration's work. The UK Cochrane Centre produces the Cochrane Library, a quarterly electronic library containing four databases: the Cochrane Database of Systematic Reviews (a rapidly expanding database of systematic reviews, regularly updated as new evidence becomes available); the Cochrane Controlled Trials Register (a register of identified trials, with titles and journal references, which might be incorporated into a systematic review); the Cochrane Review Methodology Database (containing information for those who wish to undertake research synthesis); and the Database of Abstracts of Reviews of Effectiveness (see below). The library is available on CD-ROM and on the Internet.

The other major body is the NHS Centre for Reviews and Dissemination (CRD), based at the University of York, which aims to identify and review the results of good quality health research

and to disseminate the findings to key decision makers in the NHS and to consumers of health care services. It therefore works in concert with the UK Cochrane Centre, with particular responsibility for the dissemination of its work, and with the HTA Programme (generally where HTA requires systematic review rather than original research). The CRD publishes the *Effective Health Care Bulletin* to NHS managers and senior clinicians, and the more light weight *Effectiveness Matters* to all doctors in the country.

The CRD reviews cover the effectiveness of care for particular conditions, the effectiveness of health technologies, and evidence on efficient methods of organising and delivering particular types of health care. It also creates the Database of Abstracts of Reviews of Effectiveness (DARE), a collection of records of good quality research reviews of the effectiveness of health care interventions, and the management and organisation of health services. These reviews are evaluated according to a set of quality criteria, and those of high quality are included in DARE in a structured format. Reviews that are of lower quality and a range of other abstracts of reviews are also briefly covered in DARE.

The CRD also manage the NHS Economic Evaluations database, containing abstracts of published economic evaluations of health care interventions. The record of a study will normally include a structured summary and an assessment of the quality of the studies, together with details of any practical implications for the NHS.

The NHS R&D Centre for Evidence Based Medicine, also based in Oxford, promotes understanding and training in evidence based medicine, which is the application of the results of clinical trials or systematic enquiries of the kind conducted by the other centres described. The centre also undertakes original research into the practice of evidence based medicine, for example, why doctors do not always apply the knowledge they possess, or how best to present results of studies so that they can be understood and applied more easily.

Local initiatives

There are a number of local initiatives which, because of their quality, have attracted a considerable degree of national attention; many of these again relate to other areas of medical intervention as well as drugs.

128

Development and Evaluation Committee (DEC) reports are produced as part of the Development and Evaluation Service, funded locally by the South and West NHS Executive. They are intended to provide rapid, accurate, and usable information on effectiveness of health technologies to purchasers, clinicians, managers, and researchers in the south and west of the country, but they also disseminate widely and have a much wider influence. There are two elements to the report: an expert technical report on technology and the recommendation of an independent committee (DEC), made up of senior clinicians and other experienced individuals who formally review the evidence presented, on whether the intervention should be purchased. The Public Health Resource Unit in Oxford and the Anglia Clinical Effectiveness Team provide a similar resource for Oxford and Anglia NHS R&D Directorate, and similar systems operate in other regions. In addition, Anglia and Oxford fund *Bandolier*, a monthly journal on matters of clinical effectiveness which contains bullet points of evidence based medicine (hence its title).

West Midlands health authorities fund Midland Therapeutic Review and Advisory Committee (MTRAC), which considers only drug therapies and is described fully in chapter 9.

Prescribing research

The Department of Health has funded a range of research projects looking at various aspects of prescribing, including prescribing at the interface between primary and secondary care, the effects of NHS reforms on prescribing, the effectiveness of academic detailing in the UK, and the influences on prescribing. The aim of this research is to give a better understanding of prescribing so as to enhance our ability to improve it. The results of these studies will be published over the next few years.

Other organisations promoting good medicines management

The Consumers' Association publish the *Drug and Therapeutics Bulletin*, a highly respected and influential drug information journal. It is distributed free of charge to all doctors in the UK,

funded by the Department of Health which, however, has no influence on the editorial line taken by the bulletin. The Consumers' Association also organises regular seminars on issues related to drug use.

The Drug Information Pharmacists' Group (DIPG) is a collaboration of drug information pharmacists across the UK to coordinate their efforts and avoid duplication, particularly in assessing new drugs. Independently evaluated information and advice are provided on all aspects of drug therapy. Historically, drug information pharmacists have served secondary care more than primary care, but in recent years have increasingly recognised the move to a primary care led NHS and shifted their efforts accordingly. Each Drug Information Centre will also produce local materials and will respond to local questions from health care professionals. Recently, the DIPG and the National Prescribing Centre are collaborating to produce a series of monographs on forthcoming therapies and their likely impact, aimed at NHS managers to inform them of future pressures and probable changing patterns of care. Local drug information services will also support other units already mentioned, such as the South and West DEC.

The future

One further national structure which will undoubtedly influence prescribing in the future is the National Institute for Clinical Excellence (NICE), proposed in the recent White Paper (December 1997).[1] The exact shape of this Institute and its methods of working are not yet clear, other than "that it will give a strong lead on clinical and cost effectiveness" by drawing up guidelines on disease management, and will undoubtedly strongly influence the National Service Frameworks; these will define what care and what quality of care patients can expect from the NHS across the country. The institute will probably build on existing structures, many of which are described above, rather than replace them completely. It will involve health professionals, health economists, managers, and, most important perhaps, patient interests. It is clear that appropriate prescribing and the promotion of good management of medicines will continue to be a major issue of focus for the Government.

Conclusion

- A wide range of managerial and professional and academic bodies are identified which contribute to good management of medicines within the UK.
- All of these are funded directly or indirectly by the taxpayer.
- Each organisation has a different role, and coordination and cooperation between these organisations are clearly essential.
- The new National Institute of Clinical Excellence will draw on this framework.

Some important addresses

National Prescribing Centre
The Infirmary
70 Pembroke Place
Liverpool L69 3GF
http://www.npc.co.uk/

NHS Centre for Reviews and Dissemination
University of York, York, YO1 5DD
http://nhscrd.york.ac.uk/

UK Cochrane Centre
Summertown Pavilion
Middle Way
Oxford OX2 7LG
Access to Cochrane Library
http://www.cochrane.co.uk/

Access to DARE (Database of Abstracts of Reviews of Effectiveness)
and to Economic Evaluations Database
http://nhscrd.york.ac.uk/

Prescription Pricing Authority
Bridge House
152 Pilgrim Street
Newcastle NE1 6SN
http://www.ppa.org.uk/

Development and Evaluation Service
NHS Executive South and West Research and Development
Directorate
Canynge Hall
Whiteladies Road
Clifton
Bristol BS8 2PR
http://www.soton.ac.uk/

Drug and Therapeutics Bulletin
2 Marylebone Rd
London NW1 4DF
http://www.which.net/nonsub/pubs/dtb/intro.html

Medicines Control Agency
Market Towers
1 Nine Elms Lane
London SW8 5NQ
http://www.open.gov.uk/mca/mcahome.htm

National Coordinating Centre for Health Technology
Assessment
Boldrewood
University of Southampton
Highfield
Southampton SO16 7PX
http://www.soton.ac.uk/ ~ wi/hta/

Bandolier
http://www.jr2.ox.ac.uk/bandolier/index.html

The UK Drug Information Pharmacists Group
(Addresses for local drug information services can be found in
the *British National Formulary*)
www.ukdipg.org.uk

1 Secretary of State for Health. *The new NHS.* London: The Stationery Office Ltd, 1997.
2 Sheldon T, Chalmers I. The UK Cochrane Centre and the NHS Centre for Reviews and Dissemination: respective roles within the Information Systems Strategy of the NHS R&D Programme, coordination and principles underlying collaboration. *Health Economics* 1994;3:201–3.

9 Getting research into practice

ALISON BLENKINSOPP, WENDY CLARK,
IAN PURVES, MIKE FISHER

Objectives

- To consider the barriers to evidence based prescribing change.
- To highlight the operation of a region wide, GP led prescribing committee, the Midland Therapeutic Review and Advisory Committee (MTRAC).
- To describe a computerised prescribing decision support system for primary care (PRODIGY).
- To describe the work of medical audit advisory groups (MAAGs) and their influence on primary care prescribing.
- To describe the actual and potential roles of pharmacists in helping GP practices to assess and implement evidence.

The National Health Service has established a framework for the collection and dissemination of research findings. Yet prescribing practice does not always reflect current evidence, and the lag time for the adoption and implementation of research findings has been a matter for concern. Indeed, in 1995, the NHS commissioned a programme of research and development to address this area. The reasons for the gap between research and its implementation in practice are complex.[1] The plethora of information sources and the sheer volume of information mailed to GPs may seem overwhelming. The availability of information at the point of decision making, that is, during the consultation, has been limited. It has been estimated that access to the relevant information within 30 seconds will be necessary if the consultation time is not to be lengthened. In the past it was assumed that GPs' continuing

education would enable them to make the relevant changes. A review of the effectiveness of different methods of continuing medical education showed, however, that most were relatively ineffective at achieving changes in professional practice. Provision involving *one to one* education and interactive sessions, in which physicians undertook practical activities, were found to be the most effective.[23] Research has shown that certain features of interventions are likely to enhance the uptake of evidence: ownership, relevance/applicability, credibility, and access. In this chapter, three exemplar models for achieving evidence based prescribing are presented and Table 9.1 shows their relationship with the four key features. A

Table 9.1 Exemplar interventions and their relationship to features enhancing uptake of evidence

Exemplar	Features
GP led prescribing committee (MTRAC)	Ownership, credibility, relevance
Computerised prescribing decision support system (PRODIGY)	Access, credibility
Audit of prescribing	Ownership, relevance
Educational outreach	Access, credibility, relevance

fourth model, educational outreach, is discussed in chapter 10. This chapter also considers the role of pharmacists in helping primary care prescribers to assess the research evidence and make changes.

The role of the Midland Therapeutic Review and Advisory Committee

Aims and objectives (Box 9.1)

Structure

The Midland Therapeutic Review and Advisory Committee (MTRAC) was established in the West Midlands in April 1995. It is a free standing professional committee funded by all the health authorities in the West Midlands region. The membership of MTRAC was based on that of a hospital drugs and therapeutics committee (that is, clinicians and pharmacists), but with added

Box 9.1   Aims and objectives

Aim

To provide a review system to identify the clinical value, safety, and suitability for use of pharmaceutical products in primary care, and to enable and encourage their optimum introduction in the West Midlands region.

Objectives

- To promote evidence based prescribing through an open and informed decision making process
- To give clear advice on the appropriateness of prescribing products in primary care, including treatments being transferred from secondary care, with particular focus on patient safety and good clinical practice
- To establish a system where well informed decisions on prescribing in primary care are taken by those who are responsible for prescribing and managing the costs, that is GPs
- To contribute towards the development of strategies for the equitable introduction and continued use of new treatments across the region
- To produce prescribing guidance on key policy issues in primary care and at the interface with hospital practice
- To disseminate evidence based prescribing guidance to facilitate the effective use and management of new products in primary care and at the interface with secondary care
- To define the level of partnership required to enable optimal patient care when prescribing is transferred from primary to secondary care

Table 9.2   MTRAC membership

Core members	Technical advice
GP chairman	Clinical pharmacologist
10 GPs (six attend each meeting)	Medical ethicist
Director of Public Health	Regional pharmacy adviser
Chief Executive of a health authority	Prescribing analyst
Pharmaceutical adviser of a health authority	Drug information analysts (two)
Medical adviser of a health authority	Health economist
Trust Clinical Director	

expertise from health economics, medical ethics, public health medicine, and health care management (Table 9.2). The GPs are the decision makers. The added expertise ensures that they are fully informed of both wider and specialist issues, which have implications for prescribing decisions. For example, the Committee is routinely shown all of the costs of treatment and not just the acquisition cost of the drug. The patients' perspectives can be presented by the specialist in medical ethics if the clinical evidence is ambivalent. Representation is obtained from around the region with members nominated by their local professional bodies. GP members are not required to be experts in prescribing but serve to represent the *average* GP. For this reason membership is limited to three years.

The process

Product requests

Local GPs and professional advisers identify products to be reviewed. The MTRAC office (the drug information pharmacists plus a part time secretary) also tracks major products in development that can be anticipated to have a high impact on primary care in terms of therapeutic need, company promotion (and hence patient demand) and/or cost. Thus these high profile products are considered shortly after launch.

The MTRAC also receives requests from secondary care clinicians who seek GPs to take over the prescribing of a product previously prescribed in hospital.

In the Committee's first two years to April 1997, 60 product requests have been received: 28% from general practitioners, 49% from professional advisers on behalf of GPs, 20% from the Committee, and 3% from hospital consultants.

Product evaluation

To produce prescribing guidance, the drug information pharmacists evaluate the evidence. The processes of literature searching and critical appraisal are described in chapter 5. In addition to searching the biomedical databases, the Cochrane Library, core medical journals by hand, and reference lists, the relevant pharmaceutical company is also contacted to identify any additional literature. On occasions the company will provide

136

unpublished data held as *data on file*. In a perfect world the MTRAC would wish to evaluate only data of the highest quality, that is, those obtained from comparative, randomised, controlled trials published in peer reviewed journals. For new drugs, information of this quality is usually scarce and the full range of literature has to be considered. The weaknesses, limitations, and potential biases of some literature sources used are, however, fully highlighted and considered when decisions are made.

Many new therapies are not compared, in clinical trials, against the current standard therapy, but against placebo or an old treatment option. To compensate for this, the written evaluation will often make indirect comparisons with standard care.

Thus the literature appraisal identifies the clinical value of the treatment, and highlights safety issues for use in primary care. A health economic analysis is also developed where it is relevant to do so. This appraisal is first posted to Committee members, then presented at the meeting by the drug information analyst.

Specialist advice

The literature evaluation does not give a clear indication of the practical issues of prescribing a new product, or managing patients with a particular disease/condition. To ensure that these issues are considered, and in recognition of the value of expert opinion, a specialist, who works in the area under discussion, is invited to attend to update the Committee about problems with current treatment and the potential place of the new product. The specialist clarifies the monitoring required and identifies safety issues of concern. The consultant is also willing to answer any other questions. The consultant then leaves before the discussion on whether the product should be recommended for prescription in general practice.

Decision making

The GPs focus on the practicalities of prescribing the product with particular consideration for assessment of the evidence and patient safety.

- *Efficacy*: the discussion focuses on the quality and completeness of the evidence, the novelty of the treatment, and its comparative efficacy.

- *Safety*: members consider any identified adverse effects, their complexity, and the ability of GPs to identify and manage them. Drug interactions and monitoring needs are carefully considered.
- *Support*: back up services available from specialist centres are reviewed.
- *Monitoring*: specialised screening needs are noted and the discussion focuses on the practicalities of providing them in general practice.
- *Dosage and administration issues*: unusual/unfamiliar routes of administration in general practice are noted.
- *Training needs*: the discussion identifies the need for any specialist knowledge, skills, or equipment.

Guidance

The recommendations issued by MTRAC fall within three main categories (Box 9.2).

Box 9.2   MTRAC recommendation categories

1   **Recommended**

2   **Restricted use:**
Suitable for prescription in primary care only:
(a) where back up support is available
and/or
(b) where the GP has specialist knowledge or skills in the area under consideration
and/or
(c) within the guidance of an adequate shared care arrangement

3   **Not recommended**

In the Committee's first two years, to April 1997, 41 product recommendations have been issued: 16 for new products; four for product licence changes; 18 requests from secondary care for GPs to prescribe; one for safety concerns; and two classified as *other*. The MTRAC has recommended three products for unreserved prescription, 19 for prescription with defined conditions (normally shared care agreements), and 19 have not been recommended.

The small number of products given an unrestricted recommendation may seem surprising. The reasons are briefly discussed below.

Lack of evidence of efficacy An example is anastrozole which was launched in September 1995 for the treatment of advanced breast cancer. At this time the only published literature was two abstracts. The general point is that the quality and quantity of published data to support the prescribing of new drugs need to be improved and clinical trials conducted in more representative patient groups. Routine comparisons against standard therapy are required to establish improved efficacy or safety before recommendations are made for widespread use.

Patient safety An extreme example is the received request for GPs to prescribe botulinum toxin for the treatment of blepharospasm and hemifacial spasm. The drug, which is injected subcutaneously into the muscle surrounding the eye, has serious consequences in overdose or misadministration. Not surprisingly, it was rejected for use in primary care. There are increasing requests for GPs to prescribe specialist products with potentially serious adverse effects and requiring complex monitoring. By advising against such prescribing, GPs, and, more importantly, patients are protected from harm. Our recommendations for restricted use identify the conditions required for GPs to take over the prescribing and care safely.

The need for close monitoring GPs were advised that they should only prescribe methotrexate for the treatment of rheumatoid arthritis, if they were fully conversant with such therapy and could provide the close patient monitoring required.

The need for back up support The MTRAC recommended that GPs must have a shared care agreement before prescribing tacrolimus, an immunosuppressant used in the very specialised and complex area of organ transplantation.

Training required An example of this situation is alprostadil for the treatment of impotence; GPs need to be trained on how to administer this drug and how to reverse prolonged action.

Licences GPs were advised not to prescribe unlicensed products and advised on their legal responsibilities in prescribing outside the indications of the product licence.

The outcome

The Committee's recommendations are issued as a verdict sheet for each product. This sheet shows:

- The strength of the evidence.
- Anticipated short and long term side effects.
- Any additional safety concerns.
- The cost of treatment including potential savings/increased costs.
- The recommendation.

The advice is tailored to the average GP. It is not prescriptive and does not impinge upon the doctor's right to prescribe. It is for the individual practitioner to decide whether or not to prescribe, based on the individual patient consultation, their skills, the data presented, and the local support available. The distribution list is shown as Box 9.3.

Box 9.3   Distribution list

- All GPs via their health authorities
- Professional advisers
- Local medical committees
- Directors of public health via the regional public health office
- Hospital drug and therapeutic committees
- Directors of pharmacy
- Relevant hospital specialists
- Hospital drug information pharmacists
- Others on request

In addition to the concise verdict sheet, a more detailed analysis is available for each product. This gives a fuller literature review and a summary of the health economic analysis.

Discussion

Prescribing in general, but particularly in primary care, is becoming more complex and demanding with: the increasing range and sophistication of medicines; expectations of patients; the volume of published and promotional literature; and the transfer of patient care from specialist units.

The MTRAC empowers primary care clinicians to make prescribing recommendations to their colleagues. This gives a sense of ownership that has been a hallmark of its success. A formal evaluation will be undertaken in 1998–99.

Computerised prescribing decision support (PRODIGY)

As its full title suggests, the PRODIGY project (Prescribing Rationally with Decision Support in General Practice study) aims to assist GPs in prescribing rationally through the use of a computerised decision support system.

Background

Since 1995, GPs in over 200 practices nationally have been involved in testing prototype systems designed to improve the quality of prescribing by presenting authoritative and useful clinical information to the practitioner within the consultation. PRODIGY has been a collaboration between the NHS Executive, the Sowerby Centre for Health Informatics at the University of Newcastle upon Tyne, primary care computer suppliers (AAH Meditel, EMIS, Globalsoft, MCS, Reuters), and the GPs testing the product. GPs use PRODIGY on existing clinical systems: after entry of a diagnosis the system offers clinical advice which the practitioner may use or edit. There is no erosion of clinical freedom, because the practitioner maintains complete control of diagnosis and treatment decisions. The scope of the system is ambitious, with clinical guidance covering 70% of conditions seen in general practice and PRODIGY is not restricted to drug prescribing, but deals with the full range of management issues, including referral or investigation, doctor/patient shared advice screens, and patient information leaflets. PRODIGY may also be used for educational purposes and includes background information, such as the rationale for drug choice, although this information is not routinely presented to the clinician during the consultation.

Clinical recommendations are drawn up by a multidisciplinary team, including GPs, pharmacists, and a health authority prescribing adviser, and are endorsed by an eminent validation committee. The project team carries out pioneering work towards

141

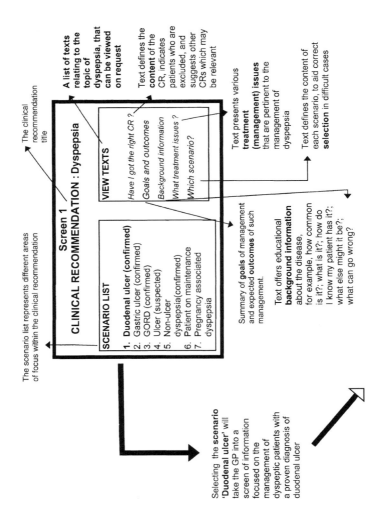

The scenario list represents different areas of focus within the clinical recommendation

The clinical recommendation title

A list of texts relating to the topic of dyspepsia, that can be viewed on request

Text defines the **content** of the CR, indicates patients who are excluded, and suggests other CRs which may be relevant

Screen 1
CLINICAL RECOMMENDATION : Dyspepsia

VIEW TEXTS

Have I got the right CR ?
Goals and outcomes
Background information
What treatment issues ?
Which scenario?

Text presents various **treatment (management) issues** that are pertinent to the management of dyspepsia

Text defines the content of each scenario, to aid correct **selection** in difficult cases

SCENARIO LIST

1. **Duodenal ulcer (confirmed)**
2. Gastric ulcer (confirmed)
3. GORD (confirmed)
4. Ulcer (suspected)
5. Non-ulcer dyspepsia(confirmed)
6. Patient on maintenance
7. Pregnancy associated dyspepsia

Summary of **goals** of management and expected **outcomes** of such management.

Text offers educational **background information** about the disease, for example, how common is it?; what is it?; how do I know my patient has it?; what else might it be?; what can go wrong?

Selecting the **scenario 'Duodenal ulcer'** will take the GP into a screen of information focused on the management of dyspeptic patients with a proven diagnosis of duodenal ulcer

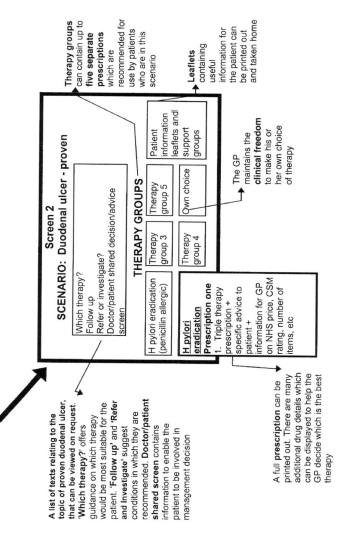

Figure 9.1 Structure of a typical PRODIGY clinical recommendation—dyspepsia
Source: Ian Purves, Sowerby Centre for Health Informatics at Newcastle upon Tyne.

developing a rigorous method for integrating evidence into rational, educational, and interventional guidelines, and methods are constantly evolving. Currently, all recommendations stem from two main sources: either existing national guidelines are adopted and adapted into PRODIGY or a clinical recommendation is developed from a full literature search and review by the PRODIGY team. Efficacy and safety are the primary considerations in therapy selection, with generic products recommended wherever possible.

GP attitudes towards computerised decision support for prescribing

A national survey carried out as part of the project research suggested that the concept of computerised decision support was highly acceptable to the primary care community, with 87% of responding GPs saying that they would like a set of high quality prescribing guidelines.[4] When asked what format these should take, 84% of the practitioners specified that the guidance should be presented on the practice computer. There was also a positive response among GPs who tested the first version of PRODIGY during 1996, with 94% of the users who completed a questionnaire considering that PRODIGY was a product worth developing.[4] The findings of the first phase of research were used to develop a second version of PRODIGY, which is currently being evaluated. Changes in the most recent system include presentation of guidance in a more structured format: after entering a problem heading, the practitioner is asked to select a scenario and then a therapy group, before being presented with a choice of prescriptions (Fig 9.1). This new structure is intended to expand the range of therapy options, without increasing the cognitive load on the practitioner.

The future

No final decision will be taken on the future of PRODIGY until evaluation is complete, although at the time of writing it is possible to state that workshop evidence suggests that GP users regard the second system as an improvement on the first. Further research is planned, with a particular focus on the complexities of chronic disease management. The team from the Sowerby Centre will also

be looking to build on existing links with other sources of prescribing support, such as the health authority prescribing advisers, in considering the way forward.

The role of clinical audit

Clinical audit is defined as "the systematic critical analysis of the quality of clinical care"[5] and has much in common with clinical quality improvement. All health professions involved with the delivery of care to individual patients are now expected to undertake regular audit, which has been a focus of attention since the 1989 NHS reforms. Audit of prescribing is one area of clinical audit that has the ability, by reviewing the literature and current practice, to introduce research evidence into practice.

Medical audit advisory groups

Audit's profile was raised significantly when legal changes were initiated in 1989 for medical audit advisory groups (MAAGs) to be set up as statutory bodies, as a subcommittee of each Family Health Service Authority.[5] MAAGs are funded by health authorities but remain *separate* in the sense that they are professionally led, maintain codes of confidentiality, and have as their clear focus improving standards of patient care. Primary care audit groups can assist health authorities in promoting and demonstrating clinical effectiveness in prescribing while retaining their professional lead and their credibility with local health care professionals. All groups have now changed their composition to include nurses, pharmacists, and other health professionals.

Their role is to facilitate audit among all colleagues in primary health care and to teach the discipline and models of audit.

The audit process

Marinker's definition is: "the attempt to improve the quality of clinical care by measuring the performance of those providing that care, by considering the performance in relation to desired standards, and by improving on this performance".[6] The audit process is usually represented as a cycle, although it has been

argued that it should be seen as a spiral because each reassessment moves the practice forward. All cycles start with the selection of an area or topic where standards of care require review and amendment. The next step is the definition of standards and criteria, based on the best available evidence. Data collection, analysis, and comparison to the standard follow. Gaps between the standard and current practice lead to the specification of necessary changes. Re-audit acts as a check both that the changes have been implemented and that patient care has improved. The essential elements of an effective audit are: a focus on standards and quality, a systematic approach, a commitment to change practice where necessary, and based on peer review.[7] Audit is most likely to succeed if practitioners see it as developmental and to do with quality assurance.

Targeting of audit

Audit should usually relate to a perceived problem in the standard of delivery of care and in the case of prescribing examples includes: to what extent are major evidence based changes implemented (for example, prescribing of aspirin in secondary prevention); are guidelines for treatment followed (for example, the British Thoracic Society's guidelines on asthma treatment); what is the level of adherence to the practice's prescribing formulary; and so on. The targeting of audit should therefore first be problem oriented, prioritised according to level of risk, and aimed to maximise the benefit both to the health professional and to the patient.[8]

Success of MAAGs in the implementation of audit

Research to date suggests that the success and effectiveness of clinical audit are variable.[9] Single topic audits on prescribing or management of a specific condition organised by MAAGs can encourage large numbers of GPs to participate and can change prescribing. A health authority wide audit of prescribing of vitamin B_{12} injections, for example,[10] resulted in an increase in the level of appropriate use from 62% to 72% at follow up. The audit process has, however, often stumbled at the stage of implementation of change. A multipractice audit of hypertension, for example, resulted in improvements in the recording of certain aspects of care but no

change in the blood pressure control of the patients. Changes that require complex cognitive processes (in this case, the practitioner's approach to hypertension management) are more difficult to effect and remain a challenge.[11] An effective system for change management must be an integral part of the audit process. Prescribing audit and educational intervention carried out by a team of a clinical pharmacist and clinical pharmacologist has been shown to produce moves to more evidence based prescribing in hypertension and asthma. Here, following the educational input and agreement on treatment approaches, the pharmacist identified patient records where changes were required and annotated them with new recommendations to be considered by the GP.[12] This translation of the evidence into suggested and targeted practical action is likely to have contributed to the higher likelihood of implementation.

Clinical audit has been shown to be most easily established in the supportive environment of a well managed organisation in which health professionals communicate well with each other and with their managers, where interpersonal and organisational relationships are friendly and open, where morale is good, and where a sense of common purpose exists. Research suggests that practices most likely to participate in and complete audits are more likely to be group practices, with modern medical record systems and demonstrating good practice (for example, the use of clinical summaries and computerised age/sex registers).[13] This is paradoxical because practices that are poorly managed are almost certainly in greater need of quality improvements and will offer greater opportunities to improve patient care. The challenge is to involve such practices in the audit process, and building on success is a key principle. The role of audit support staff is important here. A controlled trial of the use of an audit facilitator in the diagnosis and treatment of childhood asthma, for example, showed that more diagnoses of asthma were made and that the patients in the intervention practices spent fewer days in hospital.[14] The intervention was cost neutral. A small controlled study showed that primary care teams working with an audit facilitator were more likely to demonstrate a developed approach to multidisciplinary audit.[15] Evaluations of audit leave no doubt that developing and sustaining clinical audit is a substantial long term commitment which requires continuing support from the highest levels within the NHS.

The role of primary care pharmacists

Background

The 1990s have seen the development of pharmacists working with GPs and their staff on prescribing. A primary care pharmacist, is defined as "a pharmacist providing services to and/or from a GP practice including pharmaceutical advice on prescribing issues and/or pharmaceutical care to the practice's cohort of patients". This definition encompasses the models of pharmaceutical advice which have emerged in recent years (Tables 9.3 and 9.4). All have the potential to work in areas where prescribing change is needed. These appointments can be full or part time and pharmacists can be from any branch of the practice.

Table 9.3   Activities, intended outcomes, and measurement of primary care pharmacists reported in the literature. I: prescribing advice—practice policies

Activity: prescribing advice—practice policies	Intended outcomes
Proprietary to generic drug switches	Increased percentage of generic drugs prescribed and dispensed
Rationalisation of formulation or delivery systems, for example, asthma inhalers, modified release dosage forms	Increased proportions of recommended formulations and delivery systems prescribed
Formulary development	Adherence to formulary drugs
Development of guidelines	Stuctured approach to treatment
Review of repeat prescribing	Controls—checks in place
Managed introduction of new drugs and new preparations	Adherence to recommendations

Prescribing advice—prescribing policies

Here, the pharmacist uses Prescribing Analysis and Cost (PACT) data to base recommendations on practice prescribing policies.[16-18] Examples might include:

- Proprietary to generic drug switches.
- Therapeutic substitution with less costly alternatives (for example, ranitidine to cimetidine).
- Rationalisation of drug selection (for example, antibiotics).

148

Table 9.4 Activities, intended outcomes and measures II: Pharmaceutical care prescribing advice to individual patients

Level	Intended benefits	Outcome measures
Individual patient medication review Locations: GP practice, community pharmacy, domiciliary, residential, or nursing home	• Identify and resolve medication related problems (for example, side effects, interactions) • Delete unnecessary items • Recommend medication change • Recommend initiation of treatment • Recommended actions to enhance patient compliance where indicated	*From patient medical records* • Drugs prescribed • Medication related problems • Recommendations for change • Proportion of recommendations adopted by prescriber *From patients* • Satisfaction with treatment and changes • Self reported adherence
Post-hospital discharge medication review	• New treatments initiated • Deletion of discontinued or duplicate items	• Intended treatment checks using discharge medication summary and patient medical records
Pharmacist led clinics Anticoagulation control	• Achieve patients' INR* within target limits • Convenience for patients	• INR results • Patient satisfaction • Direct and indirect costs
Helicobacter pylori eradication	• Initiate *H. pylori* eradication therapy • Discontinue acid suppressant therapy where possible after eradication of *H. pylori*	*From patient's medical record* • *H. pylori* test results • Prescribing level of acid suppressant drugs
Hypertension	• Implement treatment guidelines • Action to enhance patient adherence	• Blood pressure control • Patient's self reported adherence
Migraine	• Reduce GP consultations for migraine • Review use of analgesics • Recommend prophylaxis where appropriate • Treatment recommendation for acute episodes	• Patient consultation rates • Prescribing of key drugs (PACT data or patient records)

* INR, international normalised ratio.

A focus on cost containment has been the primary driver leading GPs to accept or even seek pharmaceutical input, with an emerging theme of activity around enhancing prescribing quality. Formulary

development has thus become a core activity for many primary care pharmacists, including consideration of the place of newly introduced drugs.

General practice repeat prescribing systems have become an increasing focus for pharmacist input. The type of reviews being undertaken include:

- The process by which repeat prescriptions are ordered, authorised, and issued.
- Audit of prescribing of repeat medication in particular therapeutic areas (for example, asthma and hypertension).[12 19]
- Repeat medication at individual patient level.[20–23]

Here, the pharmacist's input begins to move to the level of individual patients.

Individual patient medication review (Table 9.4)

The review of individual patients' repeat medication usually involves the identification of particular groups of patients from the practice computer system, such as:

- Elderly patients taking four or more medicines.
- Patients taking specific drugs.

For a full review, access to the patient's medical records is needed because it allows consideration not only of the medication history, but also of the symptoms and diagnosis. This enables the review to move on from a basic consideration of a medication list that can identify potential interactions and contraindications but does not allow an assessment of the appropriateness of the medication.

Other activities at individual patient level include pharmacist led medication review clinics,[24] secondary/primary care medication coordination, and strategies to enhance patient compliance.

Effectiveness of primary care pharmacists

The role of primary care pharmacists has grown from a series of developmental rather than research projects. To date there have been no controlled trials to investigate their impact and effectiveness. There is an accumulated body of evidence in the literature which indicates that primary care pharmacists have

achieved changes in prescribing, although many projects have been relatively small and conducted over quite short timescales. The objectives set have tended to be broad in nature and more to do with developing appropriate training programmes for pharmacists and the working relationship between GP and pharmacist, although some studies have measured prescribing changes.[12 19 20] The changes implemented by pharmacists have been shown to be acceptable to patients.[25]

Funding

Some health authorities have taken a lead in developing local schemes for primary care pharmacists. Funding has sometimes been from the health authority itself, and this has tended to limit developments. In 1997 health authorities were allowed, for the first time, to top slice funding from the local prescribing budget to fund pharmacist input to repeat prescribing reviews, with the agreement of the Local Medical Committee. Some one in five health authorities took up this opportunity. Thus new or extended schemes are being run in around 25 areas. The expectation is that cost savings will make this scheme at least cost neutral and initial results will be available in mid-1998. The scheme has been continued for 1998–99.

Some practices (usually fundholders) have funded their own pharmacist on a full or part time basis and there are no data to show the extent to which this has occurred.

Conclusions

- Interventions to change practice must be themselves based on evidence of effectiveness.
- Ownership, credibility, relevance, and access are key features that enhance the uptake of research evidence.
- Harnessing information technology to provide rapid decision support at the time of consultation is well received in practice.
- Clinical audit has the potential to improve prescribing, but there is a paradox that better managed practices are more likely to participate.

- Pharmacists are increasingly working with practices to audit prescribing and implement changes.
- A portfolio of methods to get research into practice is needed because no one method can meet all needs.

1 Grol R. Beliefs and evidence in changing clinical practice. *BMJ* 1997;**315**: 418–21.
2 Davis DA. Changing physician performance—a systematic review of the effect of continuing medical education strategies. *JAMA* 1995;**274**:700–5.
3 Felch WC, Scanlon DM. Bridging the gap between research and practice—the role of continuing medical education. *JAMA* 1997;**277**:155–6.
4 Purves IN, Sowerby M. PRODIGY interim report. *J Informatics Primary Care* 1996;Sept:2–8.
5 Department of Health. *Medical audit in family practitioner services. Health circular* (FP)(90) 8. London: HMSO, 1990.
6 Marinker M (ed.). *Medical audit and general practice*, 2nd edn. London: BMJ Publications, 1995.
7 Shaw C, Costain DW. Guidelines for medical audit: seven principles. *BMJ* 1984;**299**:498–9.
8 Bater R, Presley P. *The practice audit plan: a handbook of medical audit*. Bristol: RCGP Severn Faculty, 1990.
9 Baker R *et al*. Assessing the work of medical audit advisory groups in promoting audit in general practice. *Qual Health Care* 1995;**4**:234–9.
10 Fraser RC, Farooqi A, Sorrie R. Use of vitamin B$_{12}$ in Leicestershire practices: a single topic audit led by a medical audit advisory group. *BMJ* 1995;**311**: 28–30.
11 Mashru M, Lant A. Interpractice audit of diagnosis and management of hypertension in primary care: educational intervention and review of medical records. *BMJ* 1997;**314**:942–6.
12 Wood KM, Mucklow JCM, Boath EH. Influencing prescribing in primary care: a collaboration between clinical pharmacology and clinical pharmacy. *Int J Pharm Pract* 1997;**5**:1–5.
13 Levy B, Wareham K, Cheung WY. Practice characteristics associated with audit activity: a medical audit advisory group survey. *Br J Gen Pract* 1994;**44**:311–14.
14 Bryce FP, Neville RG, Crombie IK, Clark RA, McKenzie P. Controlled trial of an audit facilitator in diagnosis and treatment of childhood asthma in general practice. *BMJ* 1995;**310**:838–42.
15 Hearnshaw HM, Baker RH, Robertson N. Multidisciplinary audit in primary healthcare teams: facilitation by audit support staff. *Qual Health Care* 1994;**3**: 164–8.
16 Burton SS, Duffus PRS, Williams A. An exploration of the role of the clinical pharmacist in general practice medicine. *Pharm J* 1995;**254**:91–3.
17 Five different models for prescribing advice in general practice (report). *Pharm J* 1997;**258**:634–5.
18 Report. *GPs and pharmacists working together*. College of Pharmacy Practice, Warwick, 1997.
19 Taylor E, Thomas G, Cantrill JA. Changes in prescribing following a pharmacist-led audit of ulcer-healing therapy in general practice. *Pharm J* 1997;**259**:R6.

20 Hulme H, Wilson J, Burrill P, Goldstein R. Rationalising repeat prescribing: general practitioners and community pharmacists working together. *Pharm J* 1996;**257**:R7.

21 Donaldson SM, Radley AS, Kendall HE. Application of a formal prescription monitoring service to community pharmacy. *Int J Pharm Pract* 1995;**3**:110–14.

22 Sykes D, Westwood P, Gilleghan J. Development of a review programme for repeat prescription medicines. *Pharm J* 1996;**256**:458–60.

23 Goodyer L, Lovejoy A, Nathan A, Warnett S. "Brown bag" medication reviews in community pharmacies. *Pharm J* 1996;**256**:723–6.

24 Macgregor SH, Hamley J, Dunbar JA, Dodd TRP, Cromarty JA. Evaluation of a primary care anticoagulant clinic managed by a pharmacist. *BMJ* 1996; **312**:560.

25 Wood KM, Boath EH, Mucklow JCM, Blenkinsopp A. Changing medication: GP and patient perspectives. *Int J Pharm Pract* 1997;**5**:230–9.

10 Educational outreach

STEPHEN CHAPMAN

Objectives

- To explain the challenges of getting evidence based medicine into practice.
- To consider the need to ensure quality of prescribing and cost minimisation of resources to sustain quality initiatives.
- To describe the development of educational outreach with examples of other programmes.
- To describe the Keele model of educational outreach— IMPACT.
- To outline the training necessary to run an IMPACT team.
- To present both quantitative and qualitative evaluations of IMPACT.

Why educational outreach?

Evidence based medicine is now widely accepted as the cornerstone of good practice in both primary and secondary care. Hospital doctors have a well established and hierarchical infrastructure in their workplace to help them ensure that their prescribing decisions are evidence based. The information provided to them is usually well filtered, the evidence deconstructed, and clear guidance provided. This guidance ranges from the prescribing policies of lead consultants, which have been agreed and refined by the hospital drugs and therapeutics committee, through to the interventions and advice of ward based clinical pharmacists.

By contrast GPs are deluged with huge amounts of information from such diverse sources as the pharmaceutical industry promotional literature and medical journals, through to Central

Government guidance such as the Standing Medical Advisory Committee (SMAC) guidelines on lipid lowering drugs.[1]

Even the most dedicated GP could not hope to be able to appraise critically all the peer group reviewed literature. Initiatives such as the Cochrane Collaboration, and the Midland Therapeutic Review and Advisory Committee (MTRAC, discussed in chapter 9) address the first part of this problem, that is, critical appraisal and systematic analysis of all trials around a particular issue. The next, and even more difficult, part of implementing such evidence is getting the information to primary care prescribers and persuading them to act on it. Unlike hospital doctors, GPs are geographically dispersed, and although some are regular attendees at postgraduate meetings, most meet relatively infrequently with their peers or other health care professionals to discuss prescribing.

Although the need to improve the quality of prescribing and to exploit the advantages that new classes of drugs offer remains paramount, a publicly funded health service has to find ways to pay for such improvement. Thus, in an increasingly cost constrained health service, it is equally important that GPs understand both the evidence for new drugs and the potential for cost containment in current prescribing.

Further mailings of written information, apart from adding to the initial problem of information overload, have been proved in the past to be ineffective.[2] The next logical step is therefore to consider direct communication—face to face interviews to present a case for making a change. The past masters at this type of communication are the pharmaceutical industry with their teams of medical representatives. History is replete with examples of one drug succeeding in the market at the expense of another as a result of shrewd marketing and skilled sales people. Why not then learn from such successful strategies and use them to implement evidence based medicine?

Early models of educational outreach

The potential for exploiting such techniques was first established in 1983 by Avorn and Soumerai, in the United States of America, using a randomised controlled trial of clinical pharmacist visits to Medicaid family doctors.[2] Having proved that such visits were more effective than traditional methods

such as mailshots, they proposed the following principles for educational outreach.[3]

- Doctors should be interviewed in their own office where they are most at ease and therefore more receptive.
- Facilitators should be well presented and well briefed.
- The messages should be concise, clear, and relevant to the prescriber.
- Prescribing messages should be supported by standardised, high quality material.
- Facilitators should aim to reach as many prescribers as possible.

These principles have subsequently been applied to medical services as diverse as blood transfusion and surgical techniques.[4]

In the UK, the first researchers to apply Avorn's work in primary care were Newton-Syms et al[5] with the Prescribing Review and Independent Drug Evaluation (PRIDE) project. One clinical pharmacist visited a stratified random sample of doctors in group practices, and supported the visits with standardised brochures and posters. Drug specific messages such as the rational selection in a therapeutic group were delivered and produced an effect when compared with controls.

The PRIDE project provided the template on which the current UK structure for employing full time prescribing advisers in a health authority is based. The principle of using face to face interviews as the medium for change is preserved, but other components such as the standardised support materials and specific messages common to all health authorities have been lost. As the role has evolved, prescribing advisers are drawn into a variety of other professional activities, which means the focus of the job moves away from practice visits. Our work in the West Midlands shows that most advisers are hard pressed to visit all their GP practices[6] once a year, which the literature suggests is insufficient to produce a change.

Avorn's vision of a *sales force for the health service* has thus been partially realised—the structures are in place, but not all of the principles are being applied. The Keele model, Independent Monitoring of Prescribing Analysis Cost Trends (IMPACT), has developed a system to work within current health service structures, and provide support to professional advisers, while closely adhering to the original principles of educational outreach.

The Keele model for educational outreach—IMPACT

The acronym IMPACT is used to give the programme a distinct image that doctors recognise and associate with independent advice. Figure 10.1 shows how IMPACT bridges the gap between the credibility of the professional adviser and the communication skills of medical representatives.

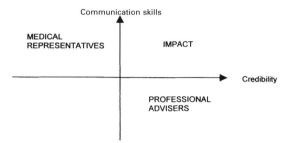

Figure 10.1   Effective Communication

Prescribing advisers have high credibility with GPs, but do not have the benefit of the extensive training in interviewing, influencing, and persuasive skills that representatives receive. In addition they do not have the time to make repeat visits on a regular basis, to be truly effective communicators. Medical representatives, in contrast, are unlikely to have a great deal of credibility, but are recruited for, and trained extensively in, influencing skills. The IMPACT model draws on the strengths of both by using community pharmacists to provide professional credibility, then training them to deliver structured messages to a timed programme.

If a health authority (HA) decides to fund an IMPACT programme it will have the following:

● Joint HA/university steering group.
● Assessment of the evidence.
● Construction of key messages.
● Design of materials.
● Specialised training programme and updates.
● Data analysis.

The programme is designed to be supportive of prescribing advisers. Health authority advisers are involved in the selection of the messages for intervention. This draws on their professional

skills and enables the intervention to move closer to a localised health authority agenda. The further element added to the IMPACT intervention programme is the provision of a field trainer to mentor and monitor the part time facilitators and provide a conduit of information for queries to and from the facilitators to the academic unit.

The steering group, comprising a GP, the health authority professional advisers, a clinical pharmacologist, a director of public health, a drug information pharmacist, and the project manager, agrees the targets, establishes appropriate communication pathways, and refines the design of the intervention programmes. The health authority decides on the topic for intervention, the university team assesses the evidence, discusses it with local experts, then constructs a package for the intervention programme.

Each potential programme is discussed with a focus group of GPs in order to incorporate their values, beliefs, and concerns in the support material. Typical programmes consist of brochures in a standardised style containing key messages, support materials such as patient information leaflets, and data analysis to show the practices with most potential for change (Fig 10.2).

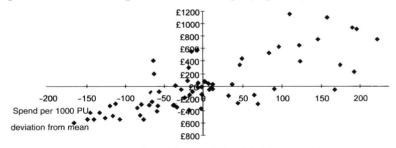

Prescriptions per 1000 PU deviation from mean

Figure 10.2   Deviation from mean spend and prescriptions for a typical health authority for antibiotics. PU, prescription unit

Selecting appropriate targets for change

The first IMPACT programme ran at a time when the drugs bill was increasing by 15% per annum, and the pressure was on to reduce costs. Potential programmes for prescribing change were therefore initially identified from aggregated Prescribing Analysis and Cost (PACT) data (see also chapter 6) as those that would

result in significant cost reduction with no reduction in quality. The selection of cost reduction targets, apart from the benefit to the NHS, meant that consequent savings were relatively easy to measure to test the effectiveness of the intervention. A selection of possible targets for change was made, some of which were known to be difficult and some to be relatively easy to achieve.

The process remains the same whether cost or quality driven. A literature search then confirms which possible changes are supported by peer reviewed evidence. Potential changes that are not so supported are rejected, as are those where the evidence is finely balanced. No more than three targeted changes are selected for each interview and, wherever possible, are linked by a common theme, for example, moving from ulcer healing drugs to gastrointestinal side effects of non-steroidal anti-inflammatory drugs (NSAIDs).

Experience has shown the initial concentration on cost reduction to be challenging and, to a certain extent, counterproductive. The success of the programme depends heavily on building good will, and purely cost reduction programmes generate a certain amount of suspicion about the independence of the advice from Central Government.

We recognise the importance of independence, as have other workers, and as we move towards quality messages, such as the use of inhaled corticosteroids for asthma or the use of lipid lowering drugs for secondary prevention of coronary heart disease, the facilitators receive a tangibly warmer response from prescribers.

Designing suitable support material

The original outreach model includes the use of standardised material. Such material, produced to a high standard, to support the campaign messages is invaluable. Not only do the brochures help give facilitators a structure to their meetings, they ensure consistency of standard and brevity, both of which prescribers appreciate. Thus when facilitators change, the consistency of the *image* of the messages helps to carry over good will.

The artwork and publishing were initially commissioned from a professional marketing agency, but as the service has developed we find it more cost effective and flexible to bring the design work *in house*. This also allows health authorities to tailor the standard

messages slightly to suit local policy, for instance on preferred regimens for *Helicobacter pylori* eradication therapy.

Other material was used to reinforce the prescribing changes in the prescriber's mind. Initially we used simple items to jog the memory such as desk pads and pens branded with the messages.

As we moved on to the quality issues we found that customised patient information leaflets for doctors to use were particularly welcomed. Our leaflets on the treatment of colds and 'flu were in great demand because prescribers used them as surrogate prescriptions instead of prescribing antibiotics to end consultations. The following year we took this one stage further by putting the same messages on buses and key billboard sites to discourage patients from visiting their doctor unnecessarily.

Recruiting and training pharmacist facilitators

Pharmacists are selected to be educational outreach facilitators when they can demonstrate good baseline knowledge of medicines and their uses. Community, rather than hospital, pharmacists are recruited because they deal with the same patient population as GPs, dispense prescriptions written by GPs, and so are familiar with their prescribing habits. In addition, because community pharmacists operate in a retail setting where informal dialogue occurs, they are also aware of patients' own expectations and concerns about their medicines.

The objective of the training programme is to move this portfolio of skills *up and across* so that they further refine their clinical and medicines knowledge, but do this in an interactive *no risk* environment where they learn to apply this knowledge using the influencing skills acquired during the programme. Clinical knowledge is updated for every new set of interventions, and influencing skills are continuously developed using the field management structure (Fig 10.3).

The following are the key attributes of the educational outreach facilitator:

- Registered pharmacist (community pharmacy practice setting).
- Technical knowledge.
- Interpersonal skills (presentation, influencing, selling, assertiveness, negotiation).
- Management skills (planning and organising).

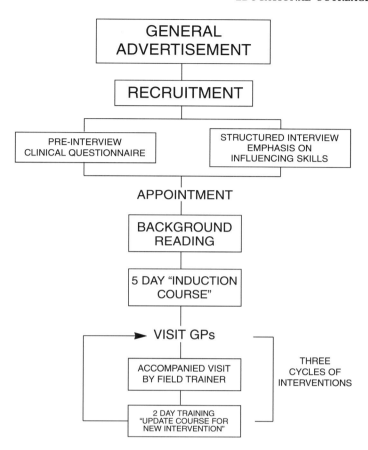

Figure 10.3   The ongoing cycle of recruitment and training (a typical one year programme)

On induction, the pharmacist participants complete a "learning styles" inventory to measure the relative preferences of individuals towards different learning styles.[7] The intention is to match the training methods of the induction programme as closely as possible to the learning style preferences of the participants. The learning styles profiles of the first cohort of pharmacists confirmed that the preselected training methods were successful. The predominant feeling from the pharmacists is that one to one training techniques, interview skills, and closing discussions are the most useful.

161

The induction training is delivered as a five day, intensive, face to face course by the department's in house team of pharmacists, clinical pharmacologist, GP, and sales trainers.

The course includes a series of assessments of both knowledge and skills. Participants are required to role play visits to the GP on a one to one basis with members of the in house training team and to present clinical papers to the group.

Pharmacists' performance in role plays and presentations is measured against a matrix of key elements of selling and presentation skills and personal qualities. Feedback is provided to participants on an individual basis and through group critiques. Knowledge is assessed through a series of written tests pre-course and at the end of the course.

In preparation for each new intervention further training is provided. The training is delivered face to face, with a focus on clinical knowledge supplemented by further videoed role play of GP visits with feedback. The average course length is two days per intervention.

The role of the field training manager

Health authorities have used several different models to provide monitoring, mentoring, and motivation following the university based training courses. Some elect to use the health authority advisers in this role, but this is time consuming and increases the pressure on, rather than supporting and freeing time for, the health authority adviser. Others have shared the cost of seconding an experienced field trainer from the pharmaceutical industry. The challenge here is maintaining independence, both real and perceived, from the sponsoring company and topics close to that company's portfolio are best avoided. Nevertheless, if managed well this model does provide the opportunity for sharing not only costs but benefits with the private sector—the health authority has a year of a seasoned trainer and the industry receives an individual more aware of the needs of the health service.

A model that works well for experienced IMPACT teams is to *upgrade* experienced facilitators by running a *train the trainers* course for them and then guiding them with ongoing support from the university base. This model, combined with update meetings, is working well.

The field training manager accompanies pharmacists on all their initial interviews and keeps in close telephone contact. Further accompanied visits are made when problems arise. Practical advice and encouragement is provided in dealing with rejections and seeking alternative strategies for unsuccessful visits.

The programme of visits to doctors

Contacting the GP practices

Pharmacists initially contact practice managers and reception staff to explain the role of IMPACT, then seek to present the intervention to all the doctors in the practice. They are encouraged to make first contact with practices in person, then follow up with telephone calls.

Telephone appointments are usually preferred. In urban areas where doctors may have no formal appointment system, less support staff, and, hence, greater time pressures, it is often difficult to make formal appointments. In these circumstances IMPACT pharmacists *cold call* to make the first contact, although subsequent visits are easier to arrange.

Each pharmacist is allocated 20–25 practices, wherever possible close to his or her home base, and is provided with a supply of programme materials, comprising written information supporting the oral message.

The university and health authority link is explained in the first visit as are the principles of educational outreach. The three targeted changes are then presented and the GPs' opinions and views sought and discussed in a non-confrontational manner. The pharmacists' training is sufficiently robust to ensure that likely objections are predicted and pharmacists have the published research papers to answer these concerns. The evidence is presented and agreement to implement change sought.

The written information is left in the surgery and copies of the key articles on which the academic message is based are offered, although these are rarely accepted. Pharmacists have the profile of local prescribing for that therapeutic area and on each visit offer to obtain and analyse that practice's prescribing. Most prescribers accept this offer.

Pharmacists are trained to be sensitive to the prescriber time pressures (and hence attention span) and the ideal interview is

conducted in 10–15 min. The objective is that each prescriber should be visited twice for each campaign and the first visit is normally closed with the invitation to obtain practice specific prescribing data or further clinical articles on the subject under discussion. On each visit the GP is invited to raise any issues of concern on other prescribing areas and these are fed back to the health authority adviser, or steering group, as appropriate.

Examples of IMPACT intervention programmes are given in Boxes 10.1–10.3.

Box 10.1   The cost-effective use of H_2-receptor antagonists and NSAIDs

Three messages are linked:

- The cost effective choice of ulcer healing agents
- Selection of NSAIDs to minimise the incidence of NSAID induced dyspepsia
- Discouragement of the use of topical NSAID formulations

The basis of these messages was cost reduction.

Box 10.2   Prescribing practice for acute treatment of infections—a reduction in volume of antibiotic prescribing

Doctors are supported by leaflets to give to patients instead of prescriptions, and by posters for the waiting room, both produced by Keele. Both explain the dangers in widespread use of antibiotics and suggest common remedies to alleviate symptoms.

Box 10.3   The use of lipid lowering drugs

The programme on lipid lowering drugs is particularly welcome to GPs and health authorities. It provides a consistent and clear approach across the authority, in line with SMAC recommendations. Data analysis shows prescribers how they compare with their peers and shows the health authority and the IMPACT team the practices where they should concentrate their messages. Distilling the guidelines into key messages and defining high risk groupings help to focus the changes needed, and the *pyramid of risk* chart provides a useful tool for discussion between doctors and also with their patients.

Data collection and analysis

User friendly reports, comparative histograms, and the prescribing matrix are supplied to each facilitator for use during their GP interviews. In this way, the pharmacist facilitators are able to focus on the clinical content and presenting their arguments well.

The advent of electronic PACT through the E-PACT system (see also chapter 6) has made the initial stages of data analysis less labour intensive and hence less costly. It is still more cost effective, however, to have data analysts undertake this part of the work than pharmacists.

Monitoring and measuring outcomes

The challenge in measuring the outcome from initiatives to promote change is separating cause and effect from the many influences that may result in a prescribing change.

For our initial research project, we used as the intervention cohort the practices that received visits. Control practices were then randomly selected from practices in the West Midlands outside the intervention health authorities.

These practices were further stratified for fundholding status and whether they were single handed or multi-partner practices. To compare *like with like*, pairs of intervention and control practices were matched for baseline prescribing. Practice level prescribing data were collected for the intervention group for three months before the intervention, the intervention period itself, and for three months afterwards. The changes in volume of prescribing were calculated using defined daily doses, as this was the WHO *gold standard* for standardised comparisons of the drugs used at the time of the project. Intervention and cohort were compared on *differences of differences* (Fig 10.4), that is, absolute drop in the median number of defined daily doses in the intervention group versus absolute drop in the median value for the control group. As the cohorts were not normally distributed, the median values were compared using a Wilcoxon matched pairs, signed ranks test.

Does IMPACT work in NHS structures?

The analysis showed that 16 of the 19 messages delivered produced a change in the desired direction.[5,7] Most of these changes

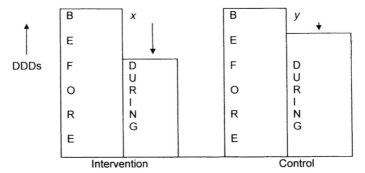

Figure 10.4   An illustration of the "differences of differences" methodology
x−y= "difference of difference"

concentrated on quality and safety issues—either avoiding adverse reactions to drugs, or preventing development of resistance to antibiotics—as well as having a cost containment perspective.

Although our primary outcome measure was the change in volume of prescribing, we did examine costs and demonstrated savings of £242 000 for two health authorities. This figure is for the duration of the active project, makes no assumption about the changes being permanent, and is likely to be a considerable underestimate.

Qualitative evaluation

An independent survey of GPs showed that they appreciated the service they received from IMPACT.[8,9] Over 80% found the facilitator's advice credible and the materials useful. When asked to score all aspects of the programme on a scale of one to five, they returned a median score of two with an interquartile range of one. Some typical quotes included:

> "He comes in, he's very focused, he gets his message across, he doesn't take too long, which means we are happy to see him regularly."
>
> "They are all very good positive messages."
>
> "Because we get information from so many sources . . . it's nice to have someone independent."

Several health authorities now routinely run IMPACT teams, and these established facilitators continue to enjoy good

relationships with prescribers, so that there is no doubt that the service is appreciated by its prime consumers. A typical programme costs the average health authority about £40 000. What IMPACT has demonstrated is that it is possible to establish a conduit of information to general practice for any prescribing message. New guidelines or drug information can be passed speedily by an IMPACT team to over 80% of practices within 12 weeks. There is still tremendous potential to use such a mechanism to ensure we promote evidence based medicine while ensuring that we offset some of the implementation costs by identification of savings.

1 Standing Medical Advisory Committee. *The use of statins*, (1106)HCD Aug 97(04). London: Department of Health, 1997.
2 Avorn J, Soumerai SB. Improving drug therapy decisions through educational outreach. *N Engl J Med* 1983;**308**:1457–63.
3 Soumerai SB, Avorn J. Principles of educational outreach (academic detailing) to improve clinical decision making. *JAMA* 1990;**263**:549–56.
4 Davis DA, Thompson MA, Oxman MD, Haynes BH. Changing physicians performance. A systematic review of continuing medical education strategies. *JAMA* 1995;**274**:700–50.
5 Newton-Syms FAO, Dawson DH, Cooke J, Feely M *et al.* The influence of an academic representative on prescribing by general practitioners. *Br J Clin Pharmacol* 1992;**33**:69–73.
6 *West Midlands Annual Report on Prescribing 1994–95*. Keele: Department of Medicines Management, Keele University, 1996.
7 Honey P, Mumford A. *The manual of learning styles*, 1986. Maidenhead, 1996.
8 Chapman S, Jones P, Earl-Slater A, Heatlie HF. Educational outreach using community pharmacists to deliver prescribing messages to general practitioners. *J Health Service Research and Policy* 1998; in press.
9 Hayes L, Blenkinsopp A. *IMPACT 2: qualitative analysis report to West Midlands NHSE*. Keele: Department of Medicines Management, Keele University, 1997.

11 Systems for controlling prescribing

RAY FITZPATRICK, NAAZ COKER

Objectives

- To review hospital structures for medicines management.
- To propose a whole systems approach to medicines management.

Background

Approximately 14% of the UK expenditure on health is spent on medicines, and considerable energy and efforts are directed at mechanisms for controlling expenditure by the Department of Health, health authorities, and Trusts. Although less than 20% of medicines expenditure is incurred in secondary care, structures and mechanisms for controlling prescribing have been developed there over the past three decades. The key driver has been cash limits in hospital medicine.

Hospital systems have been developed to produce savings, to limit choice, and to encourage appropriate use, especially by junior medical staff. Implementation and monitoring of these systems has been primarily the responsibility of hospital pharmacists, supported by drugs and therapeutics committees. These committees, which are multidisciplinary in structure, have overarching responsibility for promoting cost effective prescribing via formularies and prescribing policies.

Hospital formularies have formed the cornerstone of systems to influence the range of medicines available, whereas clinical guidelines and prescribing policies have attempted to influence choice by providing information and managing the entry of new products in to clinical practice. These approaches have been

supported by clinical pharmacy services and more recently directorate level pharmacists.

The NHS changes, which created an organisation split between purchasing and providing, resulted in health authorities employing pharmaceutical advisers to monitor and support cost effective prescribing in primary care as well as to provide a link between primary and secondary care pharmacy services. The recent Government reforms are shifting the emphasis from fragmentation to a spirit of cooperation between primary and secondary care.[1] This poses new and different challenges for medicines management and prescribing control systems.

This chapter provides a historical perspective on the development of structures and systems for controlling prescribing, reviews the strengths and constraints of the current systems, and suggests the development of a new and different approach utilising a *whole systems* approach to managing medicines. The key questions to address are:

- Why do we want to control prescribing?
- What needs controlling?
- Who can control prescribing?
- What is the system?

Formularies

These have formed the basis of the management system to control the introduction of new medicines in most hospitals for many years.[2] The concept has also been developed in primary care by using practice based formularies.[3] These can vary from a simple list of medicines with no prescribing information to a comprehensive prescribing guide. In some hospitals the list may not even be published but it is the agreed list of medicines the pharmacy stocks. The content of the formulary is usually agreed through the drugs and therapeutics committee.

The process of deciding which drugs to include should involve reviewing the evidence for clinical efficacy and cost effectiveness. In practice many inclusions are based on historical usage and reflect prescribers' consensus preference. Thus inappropriate drug choices may be given some validity and their continued use promulgated. It takes a great deal of time, however, to develop a formulary from nothing using only an evidence based approach.

A problem in implementing a formulary is to get a sense of ownership from prescribers to ensure that they adhere to the agreed choice. In hospitals this can be overcome, to some extent, by enforcing the formulary through the pharmacy and restricting access to medicines. In primary care, however, formularies have to be developed in the practice to achieve consensus. Reinforcement of changes in local formularies by community pharmacists can improve compliance with the formulary.[4]

Hospitals and health authorities perceive formularies as a way of controlling expenditure on medicines. Although it has been possible to demonstrate an impact on prescribing habits, it is very difficult to extrapolate this into savings because of the number of influencing variables, particularly the increase in numbers of patients treated. Their real strength is that they provide a basic framework for prescribing policies to be developed. They need to be flexible in order to respond to new developments and mechanisms have to be established to add or delete medicines. In so doing it is possible to introduce an evidence based approach rather than personal preference. In large organisations such as hospitals, these mechanisms need to be transparent, otherwise they have no credibility and prescribers will not use the formulary.

It could be argued that each organisation in developing its formulary is reinventing the wheel and a more efficient approach would be to have a central formulary.[5] Although the *British National Formulary* (BNF) represents what is available for prescription, the medicines listed do not consider value for money because the Medicines Control Agency (the body responsible for licensing medicines) considers only safety and efficacy. Thus, within each category, there is a range of medicines, some of which have no benefit over existing therapy but have a higher acquisition cost.

One disadvantage of a centrally produced formulary is that, as it would have to encompass the views and needs of many prescribers, it would contain a wider range of medicines than is absolutely necessary. A locally produced formulary contains a much slimmer range that more closely reflects local needs.

The answer may lie in the development of a basic skeleton formulary taking into account safety, efficacy, and value for money, which can be adapted to meet the local prescribing needs. Whatever the approach adopted, it is clear that, as evidence based practice becomes established, prescribing will also be more evidence based. A formulary is one way of achieving this.

Clinical guidelines

Formularies do not normally give any guidance on how medicines should be used and even those that give prescribing information do not place the medicine in the clinical context. Clinical guidelines seek to address this need[8] and the prescriber is given a clinical scenario and then taken through the treatment of the clinical situation in a step by step way as shown in Box 11.1.

Box 11.1   Typical format of a set of clinical guidelines

Protocol title

Description of the condition to be treated.

Recognition and assessment

This would include the key signs and symptoms of the condition, together with the recommended investigations and other conditions in which differential diagnosis is needed.

Immediate treatment

This would include any drug and non-drug treatments recommended to achieve immediate stabilisation of the condition. Any drug treatments would include details of doses, routes of administration, and duration of treatment. Alternative treatments would also be included here.

Monitoring treatment

This would outline briefly the measures used to assess the outcome of the treatment giving an indication of the frequency of any monitoring.

Subsequent management

This would give details of the recommended hospital treatment after initial stabilisation.

Discharge policy

This would describe the action in the outpatient setting with frequency of follow up appointments, recommendations to the GP, and any ongoing monitoring parameters.

In a clinical guideline the prescriber may be given preferred choices for treatment with alternatives. As they present the medicine usage in the clinical context they are more likely to influence the prescribers' therapeutic decision than a formulary alone. This approach has other advantages. It brings a degree of standardisation to treatment thus reducing the use of unfamiliar medicines and techniques, which is clearly of benefit to clinical risk management. It also means that national consensus, opinion, and guidelines can be adopted locally. This is important where medicines are being used outside their licensed indication, for example, in paediatric medicine where such prescribing is the norm. The advent of computerised prescribing in secondary care can facilitate the implementation of clinical guidelines by incorporating them into ward systems, and further steer the prescriber down a particular therapeutic path. This is useful, especially in hospitals where most prescribing on wards is undertaken by relatively inexperienced junior staff.

Clinical guidelines must be evidence based rather than promoting personal opinion. A practical difficulty is that their production is much more labour intensive than developing a formulary, because not only do they involve treatment, but also diagnosis. To date, they have only been produced for a small number of therapeutic areas. A possible disadvantage of a clinical guideline approach is that it promotes a *cookbook* mentality to therapeutics which may stifle a junior doctor's education. On the other hand, this approach may lend itself well to prescribing by other non-medical practitioners.

Clinical pharmacy

These services were developed in the UK in the late 1970s as hospital pharmacists attempted to use their knowledge of medicines to promote safe rational and economic prescribing. This role was endorsed in the health circular HC(88)54[6] and clinical pharmacy services have developed greatly over the past two decades.[7] There are three dimensions to clinical pharmacy representing a spectrum of activity:

1   The ward pharmacist reviews prescriptions for accuracy, legibility, safety, and appropriateness.

2 Clinical pharmacists are part of the prescribing team and attend ward rounds to influence therapeutic decisions at the point of prescribing.

3 Directorate pharmacists influence therapeutics at the policy making level.

Ward pharmacist

Again there is no formal evaluation of these services in the literature, but there are many case reports of therapeutic interventions by ward pharmacists, demonstrating their impact on patient care. Workload studies demonstrate the number of interventions they make. Pharmacists at ward level tend to concentrate on safety of prescriptions, either by correcting prescribing errors or by clarifying ambiguities before administration, rather than on issues of cost. The ward pharmacist does influence choice by facilitating the implementation of the formulary and in some cases by limited therapeutic substitution. The opportunity to influence choice from an economic perspective is, however, limited in a situation where the ward pharmacist is reviewing prescriptions already written.

Clinical pharmacist as part of the prescribing team

The clinical pharmacist is an integrated member of the clinical team and is in a much better position to influence therapeutic decisions, particularly on matters of cost. These pharmacists attend ward rounds, which is time consuming and may not result in many interventions. The real value, however, is that it establishes the pharmacist as a member of that team and encourages dialogue between junior doctors and pharmacists. In some specific therapeutic areas, for example, anticoagulant therapy, pharmacists have taken over prescribing and thus have full control and responsibility. The concept of other professionals undertaking prescribing has also been established with the pilot schemes for nurse prescribing in primary care.

Directorate pharmacist

An emerging area of clinical pharmacy practice is pharmacists working in clinical directorates to influence therapeutic policies.[9]

The drug budget in most hospitals has been devolved to clinical directorates, but even so expenditure on drugs continues to rise above the rate of inflation. Although much of the rise can be attributed to increased activity, clinical directorates are under increasing pressure from hospital management to review prescribing critically and hospital pharmacists are central to this task. A starting point for any discussion is the prescribing trend analysis provided by the hospital pharmacy computer system in much the same way that Prescribing Analysis and Cost (PACT) data are available in primary care. For a true picture of prescribing practice then, a more detailed drug usage review is given which examines individual patient prescriptions, matching diagnosis to therapy.[10] This is in fact a prescribing audit, particularly if there are written guidelines or prescribing policies in place. Often, as a result of such audits, policies or guidelines are developed and prescribing practice changes.

Drugs and therapeutics committees

These committees have been established in most hospitals in the UK for many years. They are the policy makers for prescribing and their role in facilitating the development of drug formularies was endorsed in the health circular HC(88)54.[6] It is surprising that their outcomes have not been rigorously evaluated, although views have been sought on their structure and value.[11]

Membership

Most of these committees are hospital based, reporting either directly, or through an executive, to Trust Management Boards and membership is now representative of the clinical directorate structure. A hospital pharmacist usually acts as secretary to the committee with a second pharmacist (drug information, clinical, or formulary management) having responsibility for a written evaluation of the evidence and in providing specialist advice.

When hospital budgets were cash limited but primary care budgets were not, hospitals considered only their drug acquisition costs and purchased at prices that they knew to be loss leading in primary care. As primary care budgets are now also cash limited and in response to pressure from health authorities, however,

hospitals are now more sensitive to primary care when making formulary decisions. This is reflected in the membership of drugs and therapeutics committees which now include health authority representatives (either medical or pharmaceutical advisers) and GPs.[12]

Role

The role of these committees is primarily developing medicine related policies and overseeing the formulary or other mechanisms to manage the introduction of new medicines. Box 11.2 shows

---

Box 11.2   Role of drugs and therapeutics committees

- Develop/approve hospital policies
- Develop/approve directorate policies
- Develop/approve nursing medicine policies
- Monitor drug budget
- Develop/approve cost containment measures
- Advise Trust of impact of new drugs
- Seek funding for new drugs
- Advise purchaser of impact of new drugs
- Seek funding from purchaser for new drugs
- Develop/approve joint treatment protocols
- Develop/approve shared care protocols
- Develop/approve patient information
- Develop/approve prescription documents
- Monitor medication errors

---

some of these. An emerging role is the development of joint treatment or shared care protocols with primary care, which are becoming increasingly important because many newer medicines are powerful and complex, and GPs require specialist advice and support in taking responsibility for prescribing them.

In most Trusts in the UK, drug budgets have been devolved to clinical directorates. It could be argued that this has reduced the need for a drugs and therapeutics committee to develop corporate prescribing policies and that individual directorates should manage

their own prescribing issues. There is indeed a more focused approach to prescribing issues at directorate level but recent evidence suggests that clinical directors welcome the independent advice and support that drugs and therapeutics committees can provide.[11] They also recognise the need for the managed introduction of new medicines. Although there has been very little critical evaluation of these committees in terms of outcome, there is a widespread perception of the benefits. Table 11.1 shows some advantages and disadvantages.

Table 11.1   Advantages and disadvantages of drugs and therapeutics committees

Advantages	Disadvantages
Body to approve policies	Conservative approach
Endorsement of pharmacy decisions	May inhibit directorate initiatives
Forum for multidisciplinary discussion	
Promote rational prescribing	Delay in being able to use new drugs
Consider corporate prescribing policies	Too restrictive
Provide independent advice	Too cost orientated
Educational role	
Promote cost containment measures	Lack of ownership by directorate
Control the introduction of new drugs	Conflict with individual clinician
Focus attention on prescribing issues	
Operate a formulary	
Liaise with primary care	
Liaison between pharmacy and clinicians	

Most committees are hospital based but there is also a need for such decision making in primary care. To meet this need there is the development of district prescribing committees with a primary care focus.[12] Reciprocal representation of Trusts will be essential if prescribing issues across the secondary/primary care interface are to be addressed.

In the West Midlands a regional primary care therapeutic review committee has been established (the Midland Therapeutic Review and Advisory Committee or MTRAC—see chapter 9). This arrangement prevents duplication of work and the potential disadvantage of an array of primary and secondary care committees each with its own perspective and conflicts of opinion.

Current status: strengths and constraints

The techniques described here have been developed over three decades, building on each other. Although each approach is complete in itself, the true benefits cannot be realised if each is applied in isolation but need to be seen in the context of the whole system. These approaches have been developed in secondary care where it is possible to apply more control. Over 80% of prescribing costs are, however, incurred in primary care where this is less easy. Thus the emphasis in medicines management in primary care has been persuasion and advice, supported by robust information systems that have embraced the concept of evidence based practice. The outcomes of prescribing control systems developing separately in primary and secondary care are that there is no cohesive approach and tensions have developed at the interface. Furthermore, the systems have been developed by health professionals for health professionals and hitherto the patients' perspective has been unheard.

Prescribing control system of the future

The health care system is changing rapidly with advances in medical technologies and biotechnologies, demographic changes, new patterns of illness with increasing focus on chronic illness, continuous innovation in treatment technologies, and rising expectations of both patients and the public for high quality services. There is new thinking about the shape of community services, which requires a fresh emphasis on primary care and different ways of supporting people with chronic illness to lead better quality lives in the community. Acute services and secondary care are being reshaped to increase specialist services and are being rationalised to improve efficiency and quality.

Furthermore, the Government's[1] emphasis on *integrated* health care services, through the establishment of locality commissioning, health action zones, and enhanced primary care groups, is more than just a structural rearrangement of services and facilities. The changes involved pose a fundamental challenge to professionals and other related providers to do different things in different ways. The implications are clear for managing medicines and developing prescribing control systems.

Medicines management has been defined as "a system that facilitates maximum benefit and minimal risk from medicines for an individual patient". For chronic disease, which is primarily managed by medicines, effective medicine management becomes even more challenging. Any control system for prescribing medicines will, however, need more than just professional knowledge. It will require the various groups of stakeholders in the system, recognising that patients are a key stakeholder group, to work together in ways whereby the diverse range of perspectives can come together for the common good.

One of the more recent authors on systems thinking and self organisation suggests that much organisational thinking is based on a mechanistic view of the world where we attempt to understand the whole by breaking it into parts.[13] What we need, it is argued, in today's complex world is to work with the whole system.

A systems approach to control of prescribing would ask:

- What is the system?
- Does it know it is a system?
- Does it have access to the intelligence that exists within the system?

A systems approach to medicines management

A systems approach allows a given situation (a system) to be viewed as a set of interacting components (subsystems) in which the relationships and interactions are as important as the components.[14] Within a system, the subsystems interact freely; actions within one system can impact and influence events in any one of the subsystems. In Fig 11.1, the system is contained within the rectangular box and the interacting subsystems are represented within the ellipses.

The secondary care provider system comprises the clinical professionals, including doctors, pharmacists, nurses, and the interacting technical and social processes in secondary care that will affect the managing of medicines.

The primary care provider system

This comprises (among others) GPs, community and practice nurses, and community pharmacists. The nature of their relationship and interaction will impact on the choice, continuation, and management of medicines for the user.

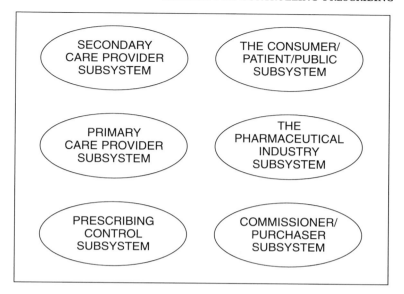

Figure 11.1   A conceptual model for a medicines management system

The consumer system

This is composed of patients and their carers, the general public, patient associations, self help groups, private health advisers, and the media. Many information tools and technologies will support and inform consumers to increase their involvement in decision making in the use of medicines.

The pharmaceutical industry system

The changing ethos of this system, from being merely product providers to becoming health care organisations, will have a significant influence on the other systems. The impact of this subsystem will, however, be determined by the nature of its relationship with the other subsystems, that is, collaborative or competitive, supportive or adversarial.

The commissioner/purchaser system

This system is set to change significantly with increased emphasis on local commissioning and the central focus on quality and

performance. Any changes in activity within this system will affect all the other subsystems and yet their outcomes cannot be predicted, resulting in an environment of continuous uncertainty and increased complexity.

The prescribing control system

This subsystem of the medicines management system, which is addressed in more detail here, is conceptualised in Fig 11.2.

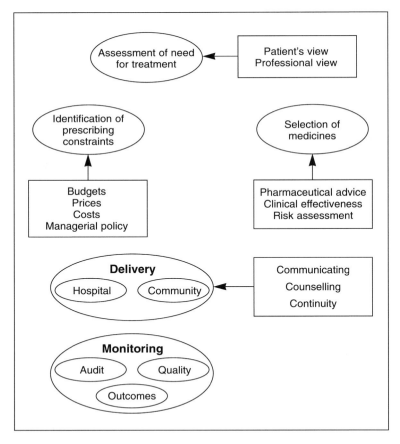

Figure 11.2   A model for a prescribing control system

This systems approach can be considered as a number of interacting processes within the subsystems such as the process of assessment of needs, identification of constraints, identification of interventions, selection of medicines, and delivery and monitoring of interventions and outcomes. Its quality will be determined by the combined qualities of the individual processes; a single process of poor quality will have a deleterious effect on the quality of the whole.

Successful management of the processes within the system requires the input of multidisciplinary teams where the potential advantages arising from the dynamics of the team are realised by fully exploiting the relationships, interactions, skills, expertise, and backgrounds of the individual members.

Factors that compromise the effectiveness of the system will need to be identified and addressed, for example, issues of interprofessional rivalries. Progress will depend on establishing a new culture and different relationships in the health system as a whole and within the components of the system.

Conclusion

A range of models and approaches has been developed over the past three decades, especially in secondary care. Although these approaches have addressed only a part of the *system* they still have much to offer. The challenge is to transfer the learning from these models into new ways of working which will address the needs of the whole system. A different framework is needed which fosters partnership, collaboration, and learning across existing and emerging professional and organisational boundaries. Thus we can mobilise creativity and improve integration of services for patients. Participation of all the key players is needed so that their range of perspectives is incorporated in service development and delivery.

Inevitably, there are significant cultural and political barriers to introducing new ways of thinking and acting. Current budgetary constraints create an added barrier to effective collaboration between primary and secondary care. This will be removed by locality purchasing.

Future steps

The following are the priorities for prescribing control in the future:

- To promote multidisciplinary responsibility and accountability.
- To consolidate and expand partnership in order to share resources and skills.
- To secure an infrastructure which allows new mechanisms for funding both locally and nationally.
- To accumulate and share knowledge and skills.
- To develop a *whole systems* approach to working.

1 Department of Health. *The new NHS: modern, dependable.* London: The Stationery Office Ltd, 1997.
2 Joshi MP, Williams A, Petrie JC. Hospital formularies in 1993: where, why and how? *Pharm J* 1994;**253**:63–5.
3 Essex B. Practice formularies: towards more rational prescribing. *BMJ* 1989; **298**:1052.
4 Ekedahl A, Petersson B, Eklund P, Rametsteiner G, Melander A. Prescribing patterns and drug costs: effects of formulary recommendations and community pharmacists information campaigns. *Int J Pharm Pract* 1994;**2**:194–8.
5 The Consumer's Association. Local drug formularies: are they worth the effort? *Drug Therapeut Bull* 1989;**27**:13–16.
6 Health Services Management. *The way forward for hospital pharmaceutical services,* HC(88)54. London: Department of Health and Social Security, 1988.
7 Boardman H, Fitzpatrick RW. *Audit of clinical pharmacy services in the West Midlands.* Report to the West Midlands Effective Medicines Unit. Keele: The Department of Medicines Management, Keele University, 1988.
8 Walshe K, Ham C. Developing clinical guidelines and protocols. In: *Acting on evidence: progress in the NHS.* Birmingham: The Health Services Management Centre, The University of Birmingham, 1997:20–21.
9 Barber N. Improving quality of drug use through hospital directorates. *Qual Health Care* 1993;**2**:3–4.
10 Cooke J. Drug utilisation research. *Int J Pharm Pract* 1991;**1**:5–9.
11 Fitzpatrick RW. Is there a place for drug and therapeutic committees in the new NHS? *Eur Hosp Pharm* 1997;**3**:143–7.
12 Wakeman A, Leach R. Joint Prescribing Committees: characteristics, progress and effectiveness. *Health Trends* 1997;**29**:52–4.
13 Wheatley MJ. *Leadership and the new science.* San Francisco: Berret-Koehler Inc. 1992.
14 Open University Business School. Systems concept and an intervention strategy. In: *Planning and managing change.* (MBA teaching material, Bill Mayon-White (ed)). Milton Keynes: The Open University Press, 1987.

12 An action plan for medicines management

RHONA PANTON

The national agenda

- Central Government needs to be sharper in defining the problems in medicines management. We all want to retain a successful drugs industry but not at the expense of jeopardising the provision of other services by prescribing drugs of little value.
- Other countries are taking more rigorous government action on price setting. Although price alone should not be the deciding factor in using medicines, the mechanism for price setting should be robust, open, and justifiable.
- The National Institute for Clinical Excellence (NICE) must develop standards for measurement of clinical and cost effectiveness and encourage national networking. It needs powers of implementation—if a drug offers clear benefit then the patient population who would benefit should be defined and funding allocated. Conversely, if a drug is not worth buying then NICE should say so and the NHS should not pay for it.
- A product licence should not be seen as the entry to a guaranteed NHS market.
- If clinical trial results are inconclusive, then the NHS should not pay for the product until further evidence is available.
- A national electronic information system to record all medicines prescribed and dispensed is urgently needed to analyse and monitor prescribing—and vital to support locality purchasing.

The local agenda

Step 1: assessing the current situation

- Are enough resources allocated to medicines management?
- Are databases used (see chapter 5) to produce trend analyses, to anticipate increased expenditure, to identify areas for improvement, and to connect prescribing to diagnosis?
- Is the evidence assessed in a critical manner (see chapter 6) and the assessments circulated to all prescribers? This is vital for good use of resources.
- Is every possible use made of national databases and of the systematic reviews available from, for example, the Cochrane Centre (see chapter 8)?

Step 2: setting standards for change

- Repeat prescribing is the largest part of the drugs bill. Colin Bradley has identified the major issue of poor control (see chapter 3). Further work with support from pharmacists and practice nurses is a strong candidate for better management of repeat prescribing.
- Developing a systems approach to prescribing (see chapter 11). A combined budget, proposed in the White Paper, December 1997, means combined responsibility in collective decisions.
- Ensuring that decisions on drug use are clear, consistent, and grounded in evidence and ethics (see chapter 2).
- Preparing cost–benefit analyses rather than considering acquisition costs only (see chapter 6).
- Better analysis of prescribing and evaluation of the evidence.
- Developing a communication strategy for patients and local media (see chapter 1).

Step 3: setting targets for change

- Enhance and reward good practice.

- Implement research findings by educational outreach (see chapter 9).
- Stop paying for drugs that are not good value for money.
- Invest in new drugs of proven value.
- Involve and inform the local community.

Index

ABOUT THE AUTHOR

Agnes Neta Buhr HEWITT was born during the great World Depression during the "Dirty Thirties." She tells her childhood memories from birth until after her wedding. She had some help from her Mother, her older sister, her brothers and gleaning information vicariously from over hearing family members talk. Mostly, she writes from memories, events she remembers even from as early as at age two. She writes about great poverty experienced by her family, about food that was mostly home-grown, about a time when there was no electricity and no plumbing in rural farming areas. She talks about how her oldest sister became converted to evangelical Christianity from which time she hoped to convert all her family to believe as she does, and the story then takes a spiritual tone. Agnes writes about her calling to be a missionary and she needed a profession to be accepted. The author also tells about a dark shadow in their home but in spite the hardships they still found time for fun, laughter and singing. Their mother was a source of great inspiration to the family in spite of her heart condition. Agnes tells about her struggles to earn high school credits until she was finally accepted at Manitoba Teachers College. She also tells about romantic relationships which failed until she met and married a widower dentist with two sons and moved to Saskatchewan. Her story is quite emotional, and you might need a tissue while reading this book. While eventually there were twelve siblings, Agnes was the SEVENTH CHILD. Her pen name is Neta Hewy.

Lightning Source UK Ltd.
Milton Keynes UK
UKHW012337250620
365566UK00005B/966